DASH Diet Hacks for Busy Professionals

How to Reduce Blood Pressure without Sacrificing Time

By

Aimee Lewis

COPYRIGHT

Disclaimer

The information presented in this book is intended to provide general guidance on the DASH Diet and related lifestyle changes. It is not a substitute for professional medical advice or treatment, and should not be used as such.

The author and publisher of this book are not responsible for any adverse effects or consequences resulting from the use of the information presented in this book. The reader assumes full responsibility for any actions taken based on the information presented in this book.

The DASH Diet and related lifestyle changes may not be suitable for everyone. It is recommended that you consult with a healthcare professional before starting any new diet or exercise program.

The author has made every effort to ensure the accuracy and completeness of the information presented in this book. However, the author and publisher are not liable for any errors or omissions, or for any damages resulting from the use of the information presented in this book.

The names of products, brands, and other entities mentioned in this book are the trademarks of their respective owners. Use of these names does not imply endorsement or affiliation.

TABLE OF CONTENT

INTRODUCTION

Are you a busy professional struggling to maintain a healthy diet amidst a hectic schedule? You're not alone. With long work hours, tight deadlines, and endless meetings, finding the time and energy to plan and prepare healthy meals can be a daunting task. But neglecting your diet can have serious consequences, particularly if you have high blood pressure.

The good news is that the DASH (Dietary Approaches to Stop Hypertension) diet offers a simple and effective way to reduce your blood pressure and improve your overall health. And the best part? It can be easily adapted to fit a busy professional's lifestyle.

In this book, we'll explore the principles of the DASH diet and offer practical tips and recipes to help you incorporate it into your daily routine. Whether you're looking for quick and easy breakfast ideas, packable lunches for work, or simple dinner recipes for busy weeknights, we've got you covered.

But first, let's take a closer look at what the DASH diet is and why it's ideal for busy professionals

What is the DASH Diet?

The DASH diet is a dietary pattern developed by the National Institutes of Health (NIH) to help lower high blood pressure, also known as hypertension. It emphasizes a balanced and nutritious diet that is rich in fruits, vegetables, whole grains, lean proteins, and low-fat dairy products, while limiting saturated and trans fats, added sugars, and sodium.

The DASH diet has been extensively studied and has been shown to lower blood pressure and reduce the risk of heart disease, stroke, and other chronic conditions. It is also a healthy and balanced diet that can benefit anyone looking to improve their overall health and well-being.

The DASH diet emphasizes cutting back on salt while consuming more nutrient-dense foods including fruits, vegetables, and whole grains.

According to research, the DASH diet is just as efficient as taking medication in lowering blood pressure by up to 12 points. The DASH diet offers several other health advantages in addition to assisting in blood pressure reduction. They consist of:

Lower cholesterol levels, reduced risk of heart disease, cancer, diabetes, and stroke, lowered risk of these diseases, prevention of osteoporosis, and assistance with weight reduction

For these reasons, anybody wishing to improve their health should consider the DASH diet.

Why was the Dash Diet Created?

Dietary Approaches to Stop Hypertension is known as DASH. During the past 50 years, the prevalence of hypertension and high blood pressure has increased in the US. The National Institutes of Health proposed funding for research that would examine the effect of food habits on blood pressure as a result of the ongoing rise in hypertension.

The National Heart, Lung and Blood Institute closely collaborated with five prominent US medical research institutions to plan and carry out "The DASH study," the largest and most comprehensive study ever carried out. The DASH trial was distinctive in that it was based on foods that the typical individual might purchase at their neighborhood grocery store, making it simple for anybody to apply.

The DASH research
The initial DASH research ran from 1993 through July 1997. Two experimental diets were compared with one control diet in the research. One of three groups was randomly chosen from among the 459 screening individuals. They were told to consume the same foods as that group for eight weeks, during which time their blood pressure would be monitored on a regular basis. Included in the two experimental groups were:

Fruits and vegetable diet, experimental diet group 1
This group was instructed to have a conventional American diet with less sweets and snacks, but a plenty of fruits and vegetables. Their magnesium and potassium levels were comparable to those of 75% of US citizens, and they had a high fiber intake.

Group 2 of the experimental diet - DASH diet.

This group was instructed to consume a lot of low-fat dairy, fruits, and vegetables. There was little fat, but a lot of protein and fiber. Magnesium, potassium, calcium, fish, poultry, whole grains, and nuts were all abundant in this diet. Red meat, sweets, and sugar-sweetened beverages were not widely consumed. (This diet includes meals that would lower blood pressure on purpose. It also included a number of foods high in antioxidants).

Control group – The Control diet
This group was instructed to eat foods that were typical of the American diet: heavy in protein and fat and low in potassium, calcium, fiber, and magnesium.

The study's DASH findings
The DASH study's findings demonstrated that dietary habits do have an impact on persons with moderate to severe hypertension. Lower blood pressure was observed in the "fruits and vegetables" group, although it was not as noticeable as it was in the DASH group. Also, even DASH group members who did not have hypertension saw a drop in blood pressure. The study also showed that within just two weeks of beginning the DASH diet, participants with hypertension in the DASH diet group had a reduction in their blood pressure.

The sodium DASH trial
The DASH sodium research, the follow-up to "The DASH trial," examined if the DASH diet might decrease blood pressure even more efficiently if it contained less salt. The "The DASH sodium study's" two primary goals were:

1. To research how the DASH diet is affected by lower sodium levels
2. To examine how the DASH diet performs at three different sodium levels

A significant study that lasted from 1997 to 1999 was the DASH sodium research. 412 adults who had stage 1 hypertension or prehypertension participated in the study. The DASH diet group and the usual American diet group were the two groups that participated (the control diet group). Three different salt amounts were included in each group's 30-day diet: 3000 mg, 2400 mg, and 1500 mg daily. Before beginning each diet, participants consumed a high-sodium control diet for two weeks, then began a randomly assigned diet for 30 days.

The DASH sodium study's findings
Both the DASH diet and the control diet were effective in lowering blood pressure at the lower salt levels, but the DASH diet's combination with low salt intake of 1500 mg per day resulted in the largest drop in blood pressure.

Researchers also suggested lowering the national daily intake for sodium as a result of the study's findings. The American Dietary Guidelines for Americans recommend consuming no more than 2300 mg of salt each day. A daily salt intake of 1500 mg is advised for those with high blood pressure.

Why the DASH Diet is Ideal for Busy Professionals

One of the great things about the DASH diet is that it can be easily adapted to fit a busy professional's lifestyle. The diet emphasizes whole, nutrient-dense foods that provide sustained energy throughout the day, making it an ideal choice for those with demanding work schedules.

In addition, the DASH diet encourages meal planning and preparation, which can help save time and money in the long run. By planning ahead and packing your own meals and snacks, you can avoid the temptation of fast food and vending machines and ensure that you have healthy options on hand when hunger strikes.

The DASH diet is also flexible and can be customized to fit your individual needs and preferences. Whether you're a vegetarian, have dietary restrictions, or simply don't like certain foods, there are plenty of DASH-friendly options that can be tailored to your tastes.

In the following chapters, we'll dive deeper into the principles of the DASH diet and offer practical tips and recipes to help you incorporate it into your busy life. So let's get started!

How to Get Started with the DASH Diet

Getting started with the DASH diet is easy, and it all starts with making simple, sustainable changes to your diet and lifestyle. Here are some tips to help you get started:

1. **Gradually increase your intake of fruits and vegetables:** Aim to include at least 5 servings of fruits and vegetables per day. This can be achieved by adding them to your meals,

snacking on them throughout the day, or blending them into smoothies.

2. **Choose whole grains:** Opt for whole grains like brown rice, quinoa, and whole wheat bread instead of refined grains like white rice and white bread.

3. **Incorporate lean proteins:** Choose lean proteins like chicken, fish, tofu, and beans, and limit red meat and processed meats.

4. **Cut back on sodium:** The DASH diet recommends limiting sodium to 2,300 milligrams per day, or 1,500 milligrams if you have high blood pressure. This can be achieved by choosing low-sodium foods and seasoning your meals with herbs and spices instead of salt.

5. **Meal prep and plan ahead:** Set aside some time each week to plan and prep your meals and snacks. This can help you avoid the temptation of fast food and vending machines and ensure that you have healthy options on hand when hunger strikes.

By incorporating these simple changes into your daily routine, you'll be well on your way to following the DASH diet and improving your overall health. In the following chapters, we'll provide more specific guidance on meal planning and preparation, as well as offer plenty of delicious and nutritious recipes to get you started.

The DASH diet is a pattern of eating that will support long-term health, not necessarily a "diet." The DASH diet is suggested by the USDA (U.S. Department of Agriculture) as "an optimum eating plan for all Americans."

The DASH diet plan, according to the National Institutes of Health, does more than just encourage healthy eating. It gives recommendations for wholesome substitutes for fast food and processed meals. Also, according to the DASH diet's developers, "the DASH diet is a well-balanced approach to eating that urges people to limit their intake of sodium (salt) and increase their consumption of calcium, magnesium, and potassium."

The DASH diet has the following traits: Less salt intake, More vitamins and minerals, More healthy fats, More fiber, Less alcohol and caffeine, Adjustable sodium and calorie intake.

Reduce your sodium consumption by following the DASH diet's dietary and sodium intake recommendations. The DASH diet's low-sodium variant permits just 1500 mg of salt per day, whereas the conventional DASH diet allows a maximum of 2300 mg. In the typical American diet, 3500 mg of salt are consumed each day.

Increased intake of vitamins and minerals: The DASH diet's abundance of fruits, vegetables, whole grains, and other whole foods will supply you with all the vitamins and minerals you need. Magnesium and potassium, two minerals that assist to decrease or improve blood pressure, are abundant in the diet.

Increasing good fats: The DASH diet strongly recommends increasing your intake of healthy fats while reducing your intake of harmful fats. Lean meats, omega-3 fatty acids from fish and shellfish, low-fat dairy, nuts, and seeds should be substituted for saturated and trans fats. By reducing bad cholesterol and raising good cholesterol, beneficial fats contribute to the improvement of our general health.

Increased fiber intake: The DASH diet advises upping your daily intake of fiber by consuming multiple portions of fruits, vegetables, and grains. This helps to lower blood pressure and keeps you feeling full. Increased fiber intake also promotes weight reduction and aids in maintaining healthy blood sugar levels.

Alcohol and caffeine use should be reduced since they have little nutritional benefit, often include a lot of sugar, and can raise blood pressure, according to the DASH diet.

Individualized calorie and sodium intake: You have the same options for your salt consumption on the DASH diet—2300 mg/day or 1500 mg/day—as you have for your calorie intake. You can select a daily calorie intake of between 1500 and 3100 on the DASH diet. Your calorie intake will vary depending on your weight, degree of exercise, if you currently have high blood pressure or wish to avoid it, etc.

You'll probably choose the lesser calorie intake if you're overweight. If you pick the greater calorie intake level, you are probably active. You will probably choose a low-sodium diet if you have high blood pressure or are at risk of developing high blood pressure owing to genetics or other factors. To determine the ideal ratio of salt and calories for you, think about seeing your doctor.

Chapter 1

Understanding the Dash Diet Food groups

The DASH diet is simple to follow since it makes use of everyday items that you can get at your neighborhood grocery shop. The DASH diet recommends serving sizes per day for each of the various dietary groups. Your daily calorie requirements will determine how many portions you should consume.

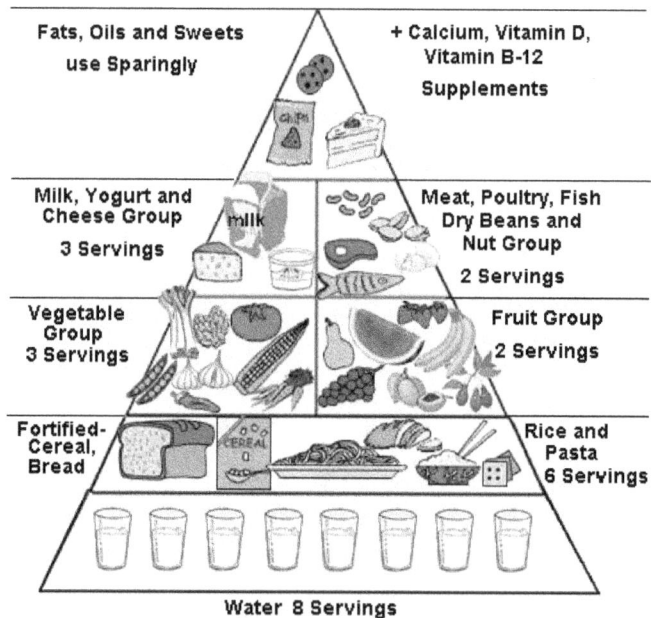

Making ensuring you acquire the appropriate nutrients should be your first goal while following any diet. Drinking adequate liquids is crucial to get the proper nutrients. Many people experience recurring cases of dehydration because they simply do not consume enough water to keep their important organs adequately hydrated.

Dehydration's dangers

Water makes up between 50 and 65 percent of the normal adult's body. Because fat tissue can not carry as much water as lean tissue, it is more difficult for your body to store the necessary water to support the appropriate functioning of your important organs when your body fat percentage increases.

You may assume that because the body has so much water already, it wouldn't require any extra, but that is untrue. As one part of the body begins to dry up, the body's overall fluid flow is reduced. In addition to slowing the blood pressure on the artery walls, this decreases blood pressure by reducing the amount of blood flow. When this occurs, there is a decrease in the amount of oxygen in the blood, which lowers the oxygen levels reaching the body's important organs and tissue. As a result of the lack of water to maintain correct fluid movement throughout your body, your entire system gradually starts to go out of balance.

How much water will you require?

Increase your fluid intake to make up for the additional fluid loss when exercising and perspiring.

To replace the fluids you lose while exercising, you should consume 4 to 8 ounces of water every fifteen minutes, followed by another 16 ounces of water.

To function properly, our bodies require 64 fluid ounces of water each day. If a nurse has ever had difficulty taking blood from you, try consuming 64 fluid ounces of water every day for a week before your blood test to see if it makes it simpler. Eight-ounce glasses of water each day are equal to 64 fluid ounces.

What to do to get the fluids you need
Although not all liquids are created equal and some might hurt your body if you drink too much of them, there are other liquids besides water that you can use to acquire fluids. Examples of liquids that might hurt your health include alcoholic beverages and sodas. On the other hand, milk is a respectable supply of fluid that can support your ability to stay hydrated. Water comes first though.

Moreover, fruits, vegetables, and the meals you consume may help you meet your water needs. For instance, watermelon, which is 90 percent water, can assist in keeping your body hydrated. Water is the main component of the DASH diet pyramid. Adding lemon and a few drops of liquid Stevia to your water is a terrific method to make it more enticing for you to drink water.

Dehydration symptoms

You become dehydrated if you wait eight hours after urinating to empty your bladder. Dark urine, fatigue, irritability, moodiness, and headaches are all indicators of dehydration. Dehydration makes it difficult for your heart to pump blood through your veins. Keep in mind that your body will respond poorly if it needs to make up for a fluid deficit.

Including a daily fluid consumption schedule

If you're anything like me, you occasionally might overlook drinking water during the day. Thankfully, there are several excellent alerts and tools available online to remind you. Avoid getting another headache over something as easy as forgetting to drink a glass of water throughout your busy day. Drink plenty of water, and your body will thank you. You'll also be lessening the strain on your heart.

Tier 2 - Fortified Cereal, Bread, Rice, Pasta

Fortified cereals, breads, rice, and pasta are included on the second layer of the DASH Diet food pyramid. This food group's whole grain types are the healthiest since they give you the most nutrients and have greater quantities of vitamins and minerals. The least quantity of processed chemicals, such as added sugars and colors, will also be present in them.

So what are the benefits of these meals for you, and how will they support your weight reduction efforts?

Energy is provided by grains.

The grainy food category helps your body maintain its level of energy when you work out or utilize your brain to solve problems, whether they be mathematical or personal.

Grain-based meals prolong your sensation of fullness.
Just adding half a cup of long grain rice to a stir-fry will help you feel fuller for longer than if you didn't eat any whole grains at all.

Oats are a fantastic source of soluble fiber, making them a fantastic choice for breakfast. The bowels become softer and are better equipped to transport your waste items along thanks to soluble fiber.

Breads operate as a bulking agent by containing insoluble fiber, which keeps your system regular.

Tier 3 - Vegetables and Fruits

In the Dash Diet Pyramid, fruits and vegetables are grouped together next. Vegetables that are more starchy fill you up more quickly and for longer periods of time.

The drawback of starchy vegetables is that they frequently contain less water than other vegetables and, when processed, turn into sugar. Avoid the error of consuming an excessive amount of starchy veggies by watching the serving sizes.

The fruit component of the DASH diet pyramid is on the other side. Fruits that are rich, sweet, and delectable might add more water to your diet. They also satisfy a natural need for sweetness that we all have.

Phytonutrients and phytochemicals are abundant in fruits and vegetables.

The vitamins and minerals found in fruits and vegetables are great for giving your body the nourishment it needs to heal itself and fight off ailments. This food group serves as your body's primary source of phytonutrients and phytochemicals.

Powerful nutrients called phytonutrients and phytochemicals shield you from conditions like hypertension as well as diabetes, stroke, heart disease, and some malignancies.

Fruits and vegetables also assist you in maintaining a healthy weight by reducing blood pressure and cholesterol levels.

Consume fruit and vegetables with color.

Consume a wide variety of colored fruits and vegetables. Imagine a rainbow. ROYGBIV is an abbreviation that might aid with rainbow color memory. This stands for all the hues of the rainbow: Red, Orange, Yellow, Green, Blue, Indigo, and Violet.

You will consume more nutrients from fruits and vegetables if their colors are more vivid and varied.

Exceeding the recommended serving size

It is preferable to eat more veggies first, then go on to fruits if you decide to consume more than the daily suggested amount, bearing in mind that some fruits will convert to sugar in your body after you eat them.

When you are deficient in a certain vitamin or mineral and there is a vegetable or fruit available that contains the exact nutrient that you need in order to correct that deficiency, adding that vegetable or fruit that you may not normally eat will allow you to cover all your nutrient bases so that you can correct your deficiency naturally rather than with a supplement.

Learn to properly prepare your fruits and veggies.
It's crucial to learn how to properly prepare fruits and vegetables so that you can get the most nutrients out of them. Fruits and vegetables might lose different amounts of nutrients throughout the cooking process.

Cooking tomatoes, for instance, differs from cooking other vegetables because tomatoes retain more nutrients the longer they are cooked. When other vegetables are cooked over extended lengths of time, the majority of their nutritional content is lost.

Vegetables lose a significant amount of their nutritional content when they are burned or cooked at high temperatures. On the other hand, after an onion or garlic clove has been diced, letting it sit for a few minutes can boost its nutritional content.

To acquire the most nutrients from the food you prepare, it's a good idea to conduct some study on the best ways to cook fruits and vegetables.

Tier 4a - Milk, Yogurt, Cheese

The milk, yogurt, and cheese categories in the DASH diet pyramid are next. It is on the same level as dry beans, nuts, fish, chicken, and dry beans.

Benefits of dairy

Dairy products are advantageous because they: Strengthen bones and teeth

aid in message transmission and reception through the nervous system

aid in relaxing and contracting muscles

aid in the body's release of hormones and other compounds aid in maintaining a regular heartbeat

Calcium is a crucial mineral that is involved in all of these biological processes. A vital component of the majority of dairy products is calcium.

Tier 4b - Fish, Poultry, Dry Beans and Nuts

The meat, poultry, fish, dry beans, eggs, and nuts category makes up the third tier of the DASH diet pyramid. This food group keeps the body healthy and strong by supplying it with protein, iron, zinc, and some vitamin B. Always pick lean cuts of meat, and skin poultry and turkey before eating.

Benefits of this category

Eggs are categorized alongside meats because they are an excellent source of protein and iron. When selecting how many eggs to eat at once, keep in mind that the yolk contains the majority of the fat in an egg.

A low-fat source of protein is beans. They also have a lot of fiber in them.

Nuts are a fantastic source of protein and iron and have a lot of healthy fat.

Tier 5 - Fats, Oils, Sweets, Supplements

The category that includes fats, oils, sweets, and supplements is at the top of the dietary pyramid. This food group's products should all be consumed in moderation. The calcium, vitamin D, vitamin B12, and supplement group is the opposite of that.

The DASH diet pyramid advises include calcium, vitamin D, and vitamin B12 in your daily routine since most individuals don't get enough of these nutrients and because we lose these vitamins as we age, making additional supplements for these particular minerals crucial.

Choose your oils and fats carefully.
It's important to pick your oils and fats intelligently. Because the body is unable to create omega-3 and omega-6 fatty acids on their own, they are referred to as "essential" fatty acids. They are only accessible through eating. These fats lessen inflammation and shield the body from cardiac problems. These fats are mostly found in fish, nuts, and several types of vegetables.
Even though processed meals have a lot of fats and oils, they are not the finest sorts to eat.

How much protein, cholesterol, and fat are permitted on the DASH diet?
Fat in total: 27%
Saturated fats: 6%

Carbohydrates - 55 % of your calories
Protein - 18 % of your calories
Cholesterol - 150 mg

Portion Control and Serving Sizes

The DASH diet places a strong emphasis on receiving the proper quantity of nutrients, eating a variety of foods, and controlling portion size. More often, it is not how much you eat rather than what you consume that is the issue.

Sure, measuring your meals to ensure that you get balanced servings of each food category throughout the day might be a hassle, but it is crucial. Thus, how can you create the habit of measuring your servings before each meal?

I long ago began dissecting store-bought packaging and discovered that I had really repackaged things in exorbitantly enormous quantities for me and my family's needed serving sizes. I would tell myself as I wrapped food that I needed to make sure I prepared enough and had enough for leftovers. After that, I began keeping an eye on what we did with the additional servings I had repackaged.

Usually, we ate more than we should have and didn't use them for what I had meant. The difference between what you truly require and what you actually consume as food is astounding. Once my husband was diagnosed with diabetes, we gradually transitioned to a new way of eating as a family. Our primary motivation for adopting new behaviors was due to his heart attack and insulin difficulties, which evolved into our food challenges.

It became crucial for me to learn how to read food packaging before making a purchase. Was the meal good enough to eat? My sense of worth abruptly transformed in what felt like a day. My understanding of the value of selecting nutrient-dense foods over those with little to no nutrients started to expand. I started portioning out snacks and putting them back into Ziploc bags. This was advantageous since you didn't have to calculate the cost of a snack. That had already been determined.

Instead of cooking extra in just one or two meals, I divided our meat packages into two, three, and even four distinct meal plans. I discovered that meals were meals and snacks were snacks. Before, my spouse would prepare a double-decker sandwich as a snack. Now that those times are in the past, we understand that a snack is just that—a nibble.

The best piece of advise I can provide is to start your "portion size repackaging efforts" with the food you already have in the cupboard, fridge, and freezer. There are a few aspects concerning serving sizes that will certainly surprise you once you start examining them. Learn about your foods and the processes taken to get them to market.

You might discover that purchasing fresh fruit and chopping it yourself encourages you to consume more of it. Why? due to the chemicals used in processing, which increase calories while decreasing portion size. Fruits that are canned frequently need sugar added as a preservation. The portion is reduced as a result.

Also, yogurt made with actual fruit will have extra additives since the maker has to do so to prevent the fruit from going bad. Often, some kind of syrup with sugar is used for this. Purchasing plain yogurt and putting your own fruit on top is a better option.

DASH diet allowable calories and servings
Fresh fruits and vegetables, low-fat dairy products, and lean forms of protein should all be a part of your daily diet, according to the DASH diet eating plan. It tries to cut back on added sugar, fats, red meat, and salt and sodium. The diet is full of potassium, magnesium, calcium, protein, and fiber, all of which help to lower blood pressure.

The suggested daily portions based on a 2,000 calorie diet are listed below. The National Institutes of Health were responsible for creating these recommendations.

Whole grains: 6 to 8 servings per day
This category includes breads, pasta, oats, cereals, rice, quinoa, rye as well as other grains. It is recommended that you choose whole grains over white and refined grains.

Sample servings:
- *1 slice bread*
- *1 ounce cereal*
- *½ cup cooked pasta or rice*

Vegetables: 4 to 6 servings per day
This category includes asparagus, broccoli, Brussels sprouts, carrots, celery, green beans, green leafy vegetables, kale, lettuce, peppers, potatoes,

pumpkin, spinach, squash, sweet potatoes, tomatoes, and turnips as well as other vegetables.

Sample servings:
> · *1 cup leafy greens*
> · *½ cup cooked or raw vegetables*
> · *½ cup vegetable juice*

Fruits: 4 to 6 servings per day
This category includes apples, bananas, cherries, dates, grapes, grapefruit, lemons, mangoes, melons, peaches, pears, pineapple, raisins, strawberries, and watermelon as well as other fruits.

Sample servings:
> · *1 medium apple, peach, or pear*
> · *½ cup fresh, frozen, or canned fruit*
> · *¼ dried fruit*

Dairy products: 2 to 3 servings per day
This category includes low-fat/nonfat milk, buttermilk, low-fat/nonfat cheeses, and low-fat/nonfat yogurt.

Sample servings:
> · *1 cup (8 ounces) milk or yogurt*
> · *1 ½ ounces cheese*

Lean protein: 3 to 6 servings per day
This category includes meats, poultry, fish, and eggs. Choose lean cuts of meat and trim away excess fat. Remove skin from poultry.
Sample servings:
> · *1 egg*
> · *1 ounce cooked meat (to visualize, 4 ounces is about the size of a deck of cards)*

Nuts, seeds, legumes: 3 to 5 servings per week

This category includes almonds, black beans, hazelnuts, kidney beans, legumes, lentils, peanuts, pumpkin seeds, split peas, and sunflower seeds as well other nuts, seeds, and legumes.

Sample servings:

> · *1/3 cup (1 ½ ounces) nuts*
> · *2 tablespoons peanut butter*
> · *2 tablespoons sunflower seeds*
> · *½ cup cooked legumes*

Fats and oils: 2-3 serving per day

This category includes coconut oil, ghee, low-fat mayonnaise, margarine, olive oil, salad dressings, and vegetable oils.

Sample servings:

> · *1 teaspoon olive oil*
> · *1 teaspoon margarine*
> · *1 tablespoons mayonnaise*
> · *2 tablespoons salad dressing*

Sweets and sugars: 5 or less per week

This category includes fruit-flavored gelatin, candy, jelly, maple syrup, sorbet, and sugar

Sample servings:

> · *1 tablespoon sugar*
> · *1 tablespoon jam*
> · *½ cup sorbet*

Dash Diet Food List

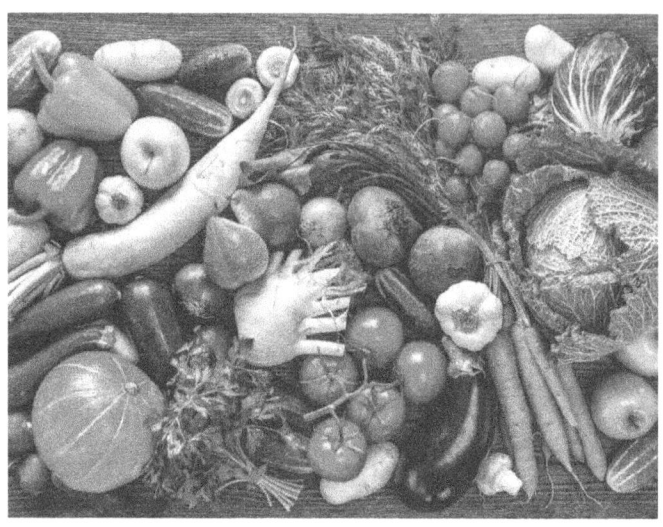

Vegetables: Low-Glycemic Vegetables (Make these your first choice)
Avocados, Arugula, Artichokes, Asparagus, Brussels, sprouts, Broccoli, Bell peppers, Celery, Cabbage, Cauliflower, Cucumbers, Collard greens, Eggplant, Green beans, Kale Lettuce (the darker the leafy green, the better), Mustard greens, Mushrooms, Onions, Radishes, Spinach, Snow peas, Swiss chard, Summer squash, Sprouts, Turnip greens, Zucchini.

Higher Glycemic Vegetables (Make these your second choice)
Butternut squash, Chickpeas, Carrots, English peas, Sweet potatoes, Spaghetti squash Tomatoes.

Not allowed
White potatoes, Corn.

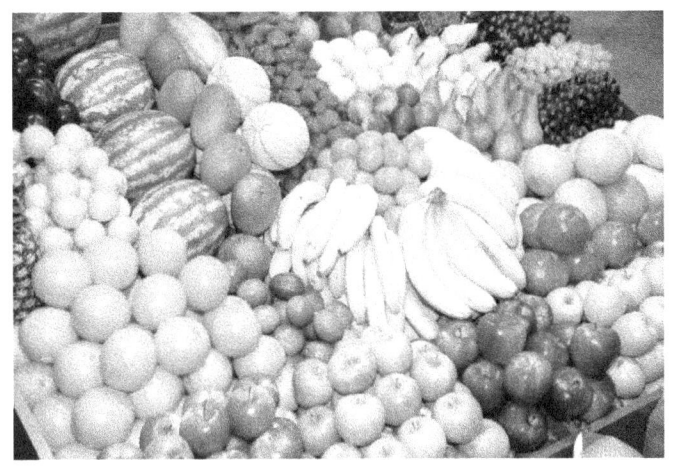

Fruits Lower: Glycemic Fruits (First choice)

All fruits are allowed, Apricots, Apples, Blackberries, Blueberries, Bananas, Cranberries, Casaba, melon, Cantaloupe, Grapes, Guavas, Honeydew, melon, Limes, Lemons, Nectarines, Peaches, Papayas, Rhubarb, Raspberries, Strawberries, Watermelons.

Higher Glycemic Fruits (Second choice)

Cherries, Figs, Grapefruits, Kiwis, Mango, Oranges, Plums, Pears, Pumpkin, Tangerines.

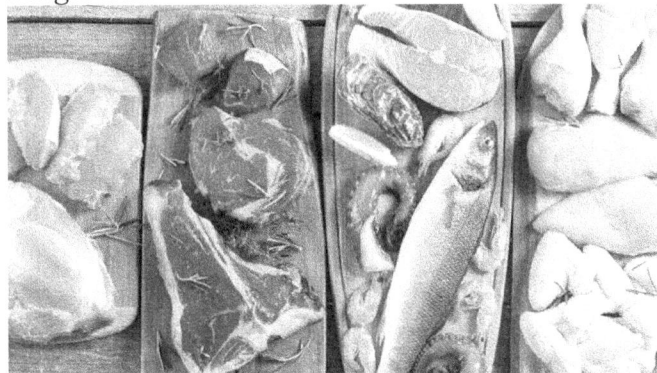

Meats and Seafood
All shellfish, All fish (especially oily fish like salmon, sardines etc), Beef (choose lean roasts and steaks and extra lean ground meat), Chicken (skinless), Eggs, Game bird, and meats, Lamb (lean), Pork (lean roasts and steaks), Turkey (skinless and ground), Turkey bacon (low sodium).

Not allowed
Bacon (regular), Cold cuts packaged and deli meats, Jerky Sausage.

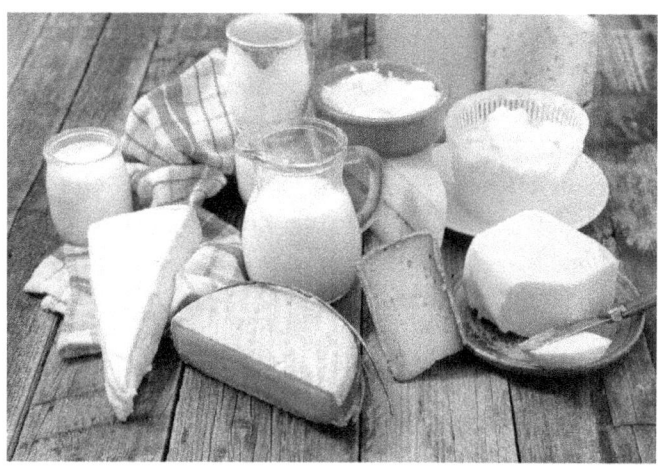

Dairy
Almond milk, Blue cheese Cheddar and cottage cheese (low-fat), Cow's milk (1 % and skim), Cream cheese (low-fat), Feta-cheese, Greek yogurt, Margarine or butter substitute, Parmesan cheese (high sodium so limit), Mozzarella cheese, Provolone cheese (low-fat), Regular yogurt (low-fat), Ricotta cheese (low-fat), Soy milk, Sour cream, (low-fat) Swiss cheese.

Not allowed

Full-fat dairy, Butter, Cream.

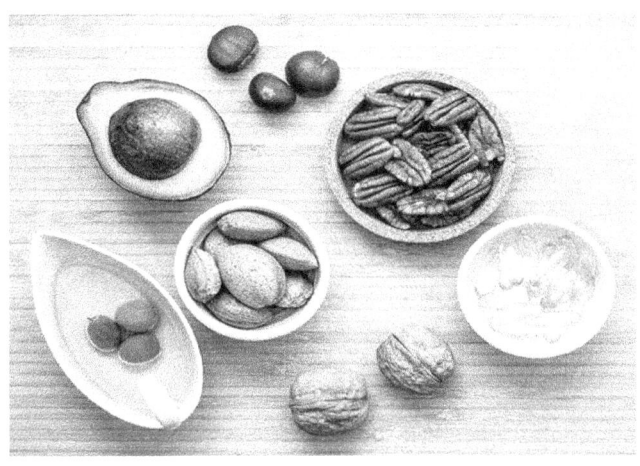

Fats
Almonds, Black walnuts, Brazil nuts, Canola oil, Flaxseed oil, Butter or Margarine substitute, Mayonnaise (low-fat), Pecans Olives (low-sodium), Olive oil, Sesame seeds, Sunflower seeds.

Not allowed
Peanut oil,
sesame oil and all other vegetable oils.

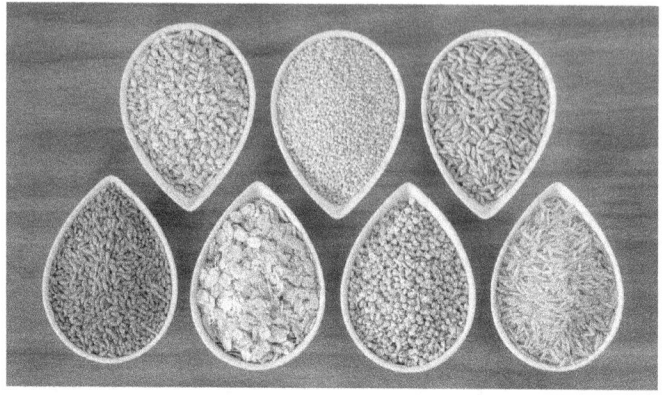

Grains

Almond flour, Brown rice, Barley, Coconut flour, Wheat germ, Whole-grain bread, Whole-grain low carb cold cereal, Whole-grain mixed grain hot cereal, Whole grain pita, Whole-grain thin bagel, Whole-grain steel-cut oats, Whole-grain thin English muffins, Whole-wheat flour, Whole-grain tortillas.

Not allowed

Corn muffins,
Corn bread,
Corn meal Oatmeal (instant or flavored),
Sweetened cold cereals.

Spices and Seasonings

It could take some getting used to going without salt if you are used to flavoring your meals with it. But don't worry; there are plenty of other approaches of enhancing the flavor of your food that don't include salting it. The fact that many herbs and spices also contain potent antioxidants and other health-boosting qualities is an added bonus. The list of herbs and spices that can be used in place of salt to flavor your meal while following the DASH diet is provided below.

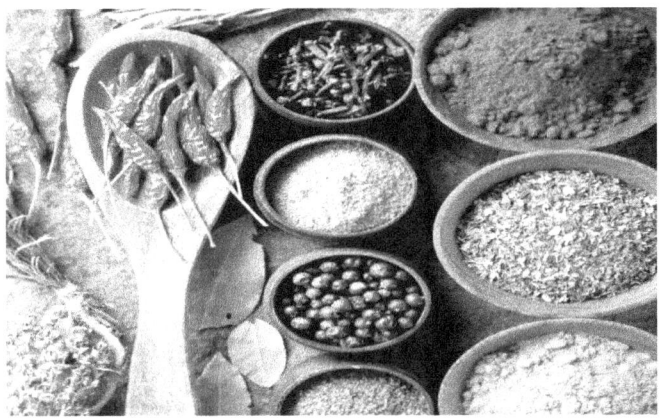

· **Basil:** *Basil is one of the most common herbs used in cooking. It has a slightly sweet and pungent taste.*
· **Bay leaves:** *These sweet and aromatic leaves are often used to enhance the flavor of meats, stews, and other dishes.*
· **Cardamom:** *Cardamom is a popular spice in Indian cooking with a peppery and citrusy taste.*
· **Cayenne:** *Cayenne has a hot and peppery flavor that will definitely spice up a dish. Also called red chili pepper.*
· **Cinnamon:** *Cinnamon can help to regulate blood sugar and lower cholesterol.*
· **Garlic/garlic powder:** *Garlic, whether fresh or in powder form, is a great alternative to salt as it not only enhances taste but has many known health-boosting properties.*
· **Ginger:** *Ginger can be used either fresh or as a powder and in addition to adding flavor has many health benefits.*

- **Lemon juice:** *A squeeze of lemon juice adds a fresh citrusy flavor that can enhance the flavor of many foods.*
- **Onion powder:** *Onion powder has a strong taste that many people love, but use sparingly or its flavor can overpower a dish.*
- **Pepper (black):** *You may think of salt and pepper as a dynamic duo but pepper is perfectly capable of standing alone. It will enhance the flavor of any dish. Choose freshly ground black pepper for a more distinct and intense taste.*

Top Hidden Sources of Sodium

You could believe that removing the salt shaker from your diet will reduce the quantity of sodium in your diet. Yet you might be shocked to realize how many items have salt buried in them. These are a few of the worst offenders.

Common Foods Include Sodium

Bread and other baked items are among the main dietary salt sources. The salt content of one slice of bread can range from 350 to 700 mg.

Carefully examine labels and select a brand with the least amount of salt. Doughnuts, muffins, and cakes prepared from baking mixes are some other baked items that are high in salt.

Cereals for breakfast: It's critical to carefully read labels since salt content in cereals vary greatly.

Sauces and condiments: The majority of store-bought sauces and condiments, including jarred spaghetti sauce, mustard, soy sauce, relish, salad dressings, and barbecue sauce, are high in salt.

Where possible, carefully read labels and choose items with little or no salt. Make your own homemade dressings and sauces for the best results.

Cheese and dairy products: are substantial sources of sodium in the diet even though most people don't associate them with salt. Salt is needed in the production of cheese. Moreover, milk has 120 mg of salt per half-cup consumption.

Foods in cans: Most canned foods, including soups, stews, and vegetables, utilize salt to taste and preserve them. The serving size in a Campbell's chicken noodle soup can contains an astounding 900 mg of salt. Also rich in salt are canned beans. Search for varieties that are low in salt and salt-free, or make your own.

Chapter 2

Quick and Easy Breakfast

Ideas

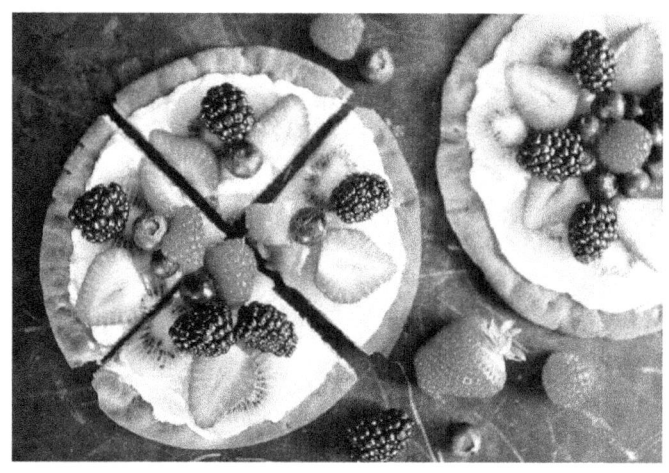

Apple-Cinnamon Baked Oatmeal

This oatmeal dish is prepared in a slow cooker so that you can easily wake up to a warm and filling breakfast.

Servings: 8

Ingredients: · *2 cups steel cut oats · 8 cups water · 1 tsp cinnamon · 1/2 tsp allspice · 1/2 tsp nutmeg · 1/4 cup brown sugar · 1 tsp vanilla extract · 2 apples, diced · 1 cup raisins · 1/2 cup unsalted, roasted walnuts, chopped*

Directions: *1. Spray slow cooker with nonstick cooking spray.*
2. Add all ingredients to slow cooker except for walnuts. Mix well to combine.
3. Set slow cooker to low setting and cook for 8 hours.
4. Serve topped with chopped walnuts

Nutritional Information (per serving)
Calories: 312
Sodium: 4 mg
Protein: 9 g
Carbs: 60 g
Fat: 7.5 g
Sugar: 23 g

Note: *To avoid a sticky mess, make sure to use steel cut oats for this recipe rather than quick or rolled oats.*

Egg White Vegetable Omelet

On the DASH diet, an omelet is a great option for breakfast, lunch, or even dinner. You can prepare a nutritious, high-protein dinner in a matter of minutes with any available vegetables.

Servings: *2*

Ingredients · *6 egg whites · 1 tablespoon water · 2 teaspoon olive oil · ½ yellow onion, chopped · 1 tomato, diced · 2-3 asparagus stalks, cut into small pieces · 3-4 mushrooms, sliced*

Directions *1 Whisk egg whites in a medium bowl, add tablespoon of water, and whisk with fork until well blended.*
2 Heat 1 teaspoon oil over medium-high heat in a medium size skillet. Add onion, tomato, asparagus, and mushrooms and sauté until vegetables are tender, about 3-4 minutes. Remove from pan and set aside.
3 Add another teaspoon of oil to the pan and allow to heat for a minute or two. Add beaten eggs to pan, tilting pan as needed so eggs cover entire pan. Let eggs set along edges of pan, this should only take a few seconds if pan is hot enough. Using spatula slide eggs away from sides of pan and tilt pan to allow more egg mixture to flow to pan surface. Repeat until eggs are almost finished, but still soft in the middle.
4 Add vegetable mixture to middle of omelet. Fold one side of omelet over toppings. Slide onto plate. Voila, it is ready to eat.

Nutritional Information (per serving)
Calories: 145
Sodium: 77 mg
Protein: 8.5 g
Carbs: 19 g
Fat: 4.5 g

Fruity Green Smoothie

This vitamin-packed smoothie is an antioxidant powerhouse, packing 2 ½ servings of fruits and veggies in each serving.

Servings: *1*

Ingredients: · *2 cups fresh spinach leaves · 1 medium banana, peeled · 7-8 strawberries, trimmed · ½ cup orange juice · 1 cup crushed ice*

Directions: *1. Place all ingredients into a blender and blend until smooth.*
2. Serve in tall glass.

Nutritional Information (per serving)
Calories: 235
Sodium: 64 mg
Protein: 5 g
Carbs: 56 g
Fat: 1.5 g
Sugar: 3.7 g

Fruit and Yogurt Breakfast Salad

The whole grains in this breakfast salad will keep you full and energized through lunch.

Servings: *6*

Ingredients: *· 2 cups water · 1/4 teaspoon salt · 3/4 cup quick cooking brown rice · 3/4 cup bulgur · 1 large apple, cored and chopped · 1 large pear, cored and chopped · 1 orange, peeled and cut into sections · 1 cup dried cranberries · 1 container (8 ounces) low-fat or nonfat Greek style yogurt, plain*

Directions: *1. Heat water in a large pot over high heat until boiling.*
2. Add in salt, rice, and bulgur. Reduce heat to low, cover, and simmer for 10 minutes. Remove from heat and let sit covered for 2 minutes.
3. Transfer grains to large bowl and refrigerate until chilled.
4. Remove chilled grains from refrigerator. Add apple, pear, oranges, and dried cranberries. Fold in yogurt and mix gently until grains and fruit are thoroughly coated.
5. Serve in bowls.

Note: *Grains can be prepared the night before and chilled overnight in the refrigerator.*

Nutritional Information (per serving)
Calories: 190
Sodium: 118 mg
Protein: 4 g
Carbs: 40 g

Fat: 1 g

Blueberry Breakfast Quinoa

Quinoa makes an excellent gluten-free alternative to oatmeal.

Servings: *4*

Ingredients: · *2 cups low-fat/nonfat milk · 1 cup quinoa, uncooked · 1/4 cup honey · 1/2 teaspoon cinnamon · 1/4 cup chopped almonds, pecans, or walnuts · 1/2 cup fresh blueberries*

Directions: *1 In a saucepan, bring milk to a low boil. Add quinoa and return to boil. Cover, reduce heat to low, and simmer until most of liquid is absorbed, about 12-15 minutes. Remove from heat. 2 Stir remaining ingredients into quinoa, cover, and allow to stand for an additional 10 minutes before serving.*

Note: *For a thinner consistency, add more milk.*

Nutritional Information (per serving)
Calories: 320
Sodium: 70 mg
Protein: 12 g
Carbs: 59 g
Fat: 5 g

Healthy Low-Fat Granola

Store-bought granola can be high in sodium and fat. Making your own is easy! Whip up a batch and store it for up to a week.

Servings: *8*

Ingredients: · *4 cups old-fashioned oats · 1/4 cup flax seed · 1/4 cup wheat germ · 1/4 cup coconut flakes · 1/4 cup pumpkin or sunflower seeds · 1/4 sliced almonds · 1/3 cup maple syrup · 1/4 cup apple juice · 1 teaspoon cinnamon · 1 teaspoon vanilla · 1/4 teaspoon salt*

Directions: *1. Preheat oven to 325 degrees F.*
2. In a large bowl, combine all ingredients. Stir well to thoroughly coat all ingredients.
3. Line rimmed cookie sheet with parchment paper. Spread mixture evenly on cookie sheet.
4. Bake in oven for 30-35 minutes, stirring once, until lightly browned.

Nutritional Information (per serving)
Calories: 180
Sodium: 85 mg
Protein: 5 g
Carbs: 30.5 g
Fat: 5.2 g

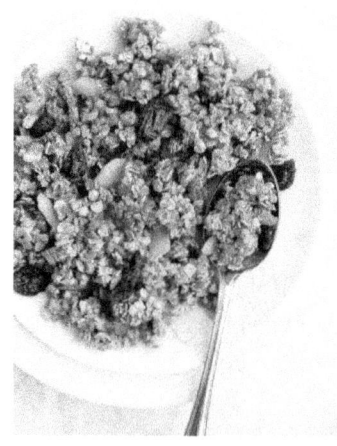

Greek Yogurt Parfait Servings

Servings: 1

Ingredients:
1/2 cup plain nonfat Greek yogurt
1/2 cup fresh berries
1/4 cup granola
1 tablespoon honey

Directions:
1. Layer the Greek yogurt, fresh berries, and granola in a glass or bowl.
2. Drizzle with honey.
3. Serve cold.

Nutritional information per serving:
Calories: 250
Protein: 19g
Fat: 3g
Carbohydrates: 43g
Fiber: 6g
Sodium: 85mg

Breakfast Burrito

Servings: *2*

Ingredients:
2 whole wheat tortillas
4 eggs
1/4 cup chopped onion
1/4 cup chopped bell pepper
1/4 cup chopped mushrooms
1/4 cup shredded low-fat cheddar cheese
Salt and pepper to taste

Directions:
1. Heat a nonstick skillet over medium heat.
2. Add the onions, bell peppers, and mushrooms and sauté until the vegetables are tender.
3. Beat the eggs in a small bowl and pour into the skillet.
4. Scramble the eggs until cooked through.
5. Warm the tortillas in a microwave or on a skillet.
6. Divide the scrambled eggs between the tortillas.
7. Sprinkle with shredded cheddar cheese.
8. Roll up the tortillas and serve hot.

Nutritional information per serving:
Calories: 300
Protein: 21g
Fat: 14g
Carbohydrates: 25g
Fiber: 6g
Sodium: 435mg

Breakfast Smoothie

Servings: *1*

Ingredients:
1/2 cup plain nonfat Greek yogurt
1/2 cup unsweetened almond milk
1/2 cup frozen berries
1/2 banana
1 tablespoon ground flaxseed

Directions:
1. Combine all ingredients in a blender.
2. Blend until smooth.
3. Serve cold.

Nutritional information per serving:

Calories: 230
Protein: 18g
Fat: 6g
Carbohydrates: 31g
Fiber: 8g
Sodium: 150mg

Veggie and Cheese Omelette

Servings: *1*

Ingredients:

2 eggs
1/4 cup chopped onion
1/4 cup chopped bell pepper
1/4 cup chopped mushrooms
1/4 cup shredded low-fat cheddar cheese
1 tablespoon olive oil
Salt and pepper to taste

Directions:

1. Heat the olive oil in a nonstick skillet over medium heat.
2. Add the onions, bell peppers, and mushrooms and sauté until the vegetables are tender.
3. Beat the eggs in a small bowl.
4. Pour the eggs into the skillet.
5. Cook until the eggs begin to set.
6. Add the shredded cheddar cheese to one side of the omelette.
7. Use a spatula to fold the other side of the omelette over the cheese.
8. Cook until the cheese is melted and the eggs are cooked through.
9. Season with salt and pepper to taste. Serve hot.

Nutritional information per serving:
Calories: 330
Protein: 24g
Fat: 23g
Carbohydrates: 7g
Fiber: 1g
Sodium: 385mg

Apple Cinnamon Pancakes

Servings: *2*

Ingredients:
1 cup whole wheat pancake mix
1/2 cup unsweetened applesauce
1/2 cup unsweetened almond milk
1 egg
1/2 teaspoon cinnamon
1/4 teaspoon nutmeg

Directions:
1. Combine all ingredients in a medium bowl.
2. Mix until just combined.
3. Heat a nonstick skillet over medium heat.
4. Pour 1/4 cup batter onto the skillet for each pancake.
5. Cook until the edges are set and bubbles form on the surface of the pancake.
6. Flip the pancake and cook for an additional 1-2 minutes.
7. Serve hot.
8.

Nutritional information per serving:
Calories: 240
Protein: 8g
Fat: 7g
Carbohydrates: 38g

Fiber: 6g
Sodium: 455mg

Veggie and Egg Scramble

Servings: *2*

Ingredients:
4 eggs
1/4 cup chopped onion
1/4 cup chopped bell pepper
1/4 cup chopped mushrooms
1 tablespoon olive oil
Salt and pepper to taste

Directions:
1. Heat the olive oil in a nonstick skillet over medium heat.
2. Add the onions, bell peppers, and mushrooms and sauté until the vegetables are tender.
3. Beat the eggs in a small bowl and pour into the skillet.
4. Scramble the eggs until cooked through.
5. Season with salt and pepper to taste.
6. Serve hot.

Nutritional information per serving:
Calories: 235
Protein: 16g
Fat: 17g
Carbohydrates: 4g
Fiber: 1g
Sodium: 210mg

Greek Yogurt Parfait

Servings: *1*

Ingredients:

1 cup nonfat Greek yogurt
1/2 cup fresh berries
1/4 cup chopped nuts
1 tablespoon honey

Directions:
Layer the Greek yogurt, fresh berries, and chopped nuts in a bowl or parfait glass.
Drizzle with honey.
Serve cold.

Nutritional information per serving:
Calories: 340
Protein: 23g
Fat: 13g
Carbohydrates: 36g
Fiber: 6g
Sodium: 70mg

Oatmeal with Fruit and Nuts

Servings: 2

Ingredients:
1 cup rolled oats
2 cups water
1/2 cup chopped fruit (such as apples, bananas, or berries)
1/4 cup chopped nuts (such as almonds or walnuts)
1 tablespoon honey

Directions:
1. Bring the rolled oats and water to a boil in a medium saucepan.

2. Reduce heat and simmer for 5-10 minutes, stirring occasionally, until the oatmeal is thick and creamy.
3. Divide the oatmeal between two bowls.
4. Top with chopped fruit, chopped nuts, and honey. Serve hot.

Nutritional information per serving:
Calories: 295
Protein: 9g
Fat: 13g
Carbohydrates: 38g
Fiber: 6g
Sodium: 0mg

Avocado Toast with Egg

Servings: *1*

Ingredients:
1 slice whole grain bread
1/4 avocado, mashed
1 egg
Salt and pepper to taste

Directions:
1. Toast the bread.
2. Spread the mashed avocado on the toast.
3. Fry or scramble the egg in a nonstick skillet.
4. Place the egg on top of the avocado toast. Season with salt and pepper to taste.
5. Serve hot.

Nutritional information per serving:
Calories: 275
Protein: 12g

Fat: 17g
Carbohydrates: 18g
Fiber: 6g
Sodium: 155mg

Greek-Style Breakfast Scramble

Servings: *1*

Ingredients:
Nonstick cooking spray
1 cup fresh spinach, chopped
1/2 cup mushrooms, chopped
1/4 onion, chopped
1 whole egg and 2 egg whites
2 tablespoons feta cheese
Freshly ground black pepper, to taste

Directions:
1. Heat a nonstick skillet over medium heat. Spray with cooking spray and add spinach, mushrooms, and onion. Sauté for 2-3 minutes until onions turn translucent and spinach has wilted.
2. Meanwhile, whisk egg and egg whites together in a bowl. Add feta cheese and pepper.
3. Pour egg mixture over vegetables. Cook eggs, stirring with spatula, for 3- 4 minutes, or until eggs are cooked through.
4. Serve hot.

Nutritional Information (per serving)
Calories: 150
Sodium: 440 mg
Protein: 17 g
Carbs: 6 g
Fat: 7 g

Spiced Pumpkin Pancakes

Servings: *10 (2 pancakes per serving)*

Ingredients:
2 cups whole wheat flour
2 teaspoons baking powder
1 teaspoon baking soda
1 teaspoon cinnamon
1/2 teaspoon ground nutmeg
1/2 teaspoon ground ginger
1/4 cup brown sugar · 1 egg yolk
1 cup canned pumpkin
2 tablespoons coconut oil · 2 cups skim milk ·
2 egg whites

Directions:
1. In a mixing bowl, combine together flour, baking powder, baking soda, cinnamon, nutmeg, and ginger.
2. In another bowl, mix together brown sugar, egg yolk, pumpkin, and coconut oil. Stir in milk.
3. Pour milk mixture into bowl with dry ingredients and stir until just combined. Do not over stir.
4. Beat egg whites in a bowl until fluffy. Fold egg whites into pancake batter.
5. Heat a nonstick griddle or large skillet over medium high heat. Spray with nonstick cooking spray.
6. When griddle is hot, ladle batter by 1/4 cup amounts onto pan. Cook until batter starts to bubble, flip, and cook until lightly browned.

Nutritional Information (per serving)
Calories: 150
Sodium: 360 mg

Protein: 6.6 g
Carbs: 32 g
Fat: 2 g

Lemon-Zucchini Muffins

Servings: *12 muffins*

Ingredients:
2 cups all-purpose flour
1/2 cup sugar
1 tablespoon baking powder
1/4 teaspoon salt
1/4 teaspoon cinnamon
1/4 teaspoon nutmeg
1 cup shredded zucchini
3/4 cup nonfat milk
2 tablespoons olive oil
2 tablespoons lemon juice
1 egg
Nonstick cooking spray

Directions:
1. Preheat oven to 400 degrees F. Prepare muffin tin by spraying lightly with cooking spray or lining with muffin liners.
2. In a mixing bowl, combine flour, sugar, baking powder, salt, cinnamon, and nutmeg.
3. In a separate bowl, combine zucchini, milk, oil, lemon juice, and egg. Stir well.
4. Add zucchini mixture to flour mixture. Stir until just combined. Do not over stir.
5. Pour batter into prepared muffin cups. Bake for 20 minutes or until light golden brown.

Nutritional Information (per serving)

Calories: 145
Sodium: 62 mg
Protein: 3 g
Carbs: 25 g
Fat: 4 g

Simple recipes for a healthy breakfast on the go

Greek Yogurt and Fruit: Mix together a single-serving container of plain Greek yogurt with your favorite chopped fruit, such as strawberries or blueberries. Add a drizzle of honey or sprinkle of granola for extra flavor and crunch.

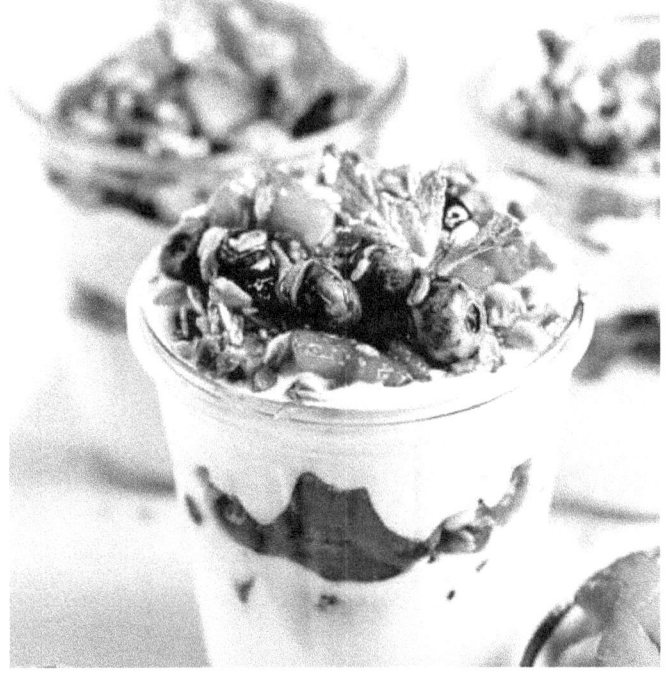

Hard-Boiled Eggs and Veggies: Boil a few eggs at the beginning of the week and pair them with raw veggies, such as carrot sticks or snap peas, for a protein-packed breakfast that you can grab and go.

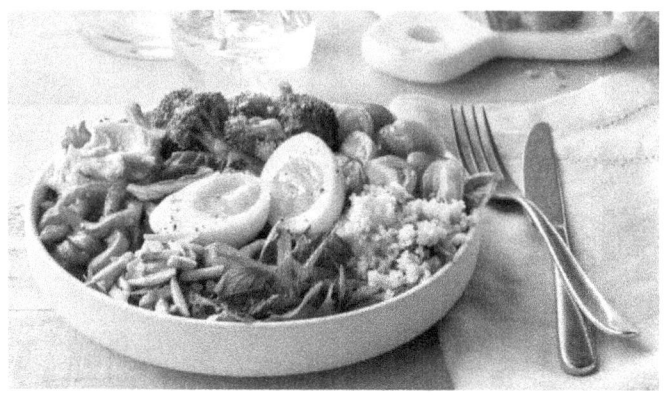

Nut Butter and Banana Wrap: Spread your favorite nut butter on a whole wheat tortilla, then top with sliced banana. Roll up the tortilla and wrap it in aluminum foil for a mess-free breakfast you can eat on the go.

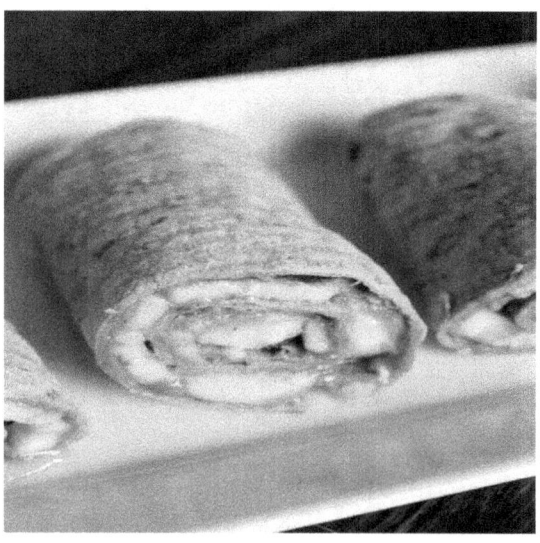

Overnight Oats: *Combine rolled oats with milk or yogurt and your choice of toppings, such as nuts or fresh fruit, in a mason jar. Let the mixture sit in the fridge overnight, then grab it and go in the morning.*

Smoothie: *Blend together your favorite fruits, a handful of spinach or kale, and a scoop of protein powder or nut butter for a quick and nutritious breakfast smoothie. Pour the smoothie into a travel cup with a lid and straw for easy sipping on the go.*

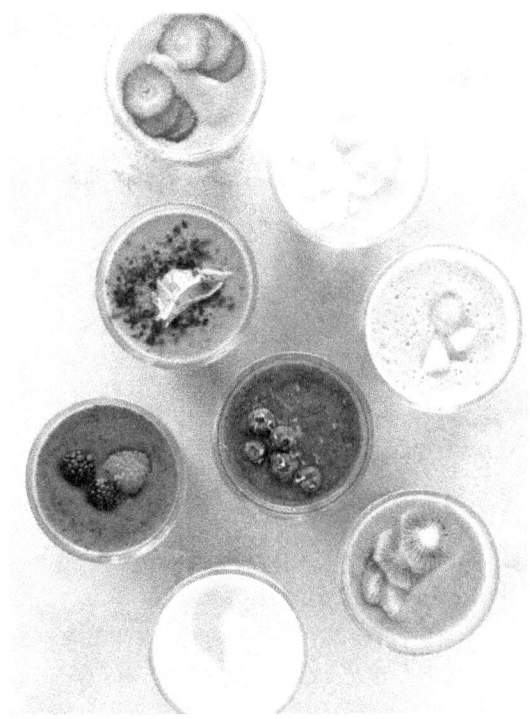

Chapter 3

Packable Lunches for Busy Professionals

Greek Pasta Salad

Servings: *4*

Ingredients:
8 oz. whole wheat penne pasta
2 cups cherry tomatoes, halved
1 cup cucumber, diced
1/2 cup red onion, diced
1/4 cup kalamata olives, pitted and chopped
1/4 cup crumbled feta cheese
1/4 cup extra-virgin olive oil
2 tbsp red wine vinegar
2 cloves garlic, minced
1/2 tsp dried oregano
Salt and pepper to taste

Directions:
1. Cook pasta according to package directions until al dente. Drain and rinse under cold water.
2. In a large bowl, combine cooked pasta, cherry tomatoes, cucumber, red onion, olives, and feta cheese.
3. In a small bowl, whisk together olive oil, red wine vinegar, garlic, oregano, salt, and pepper.
4. Pour the dressing over the pasta salad and toss to combine.

5. *Divide the pasta salad into 4 containers and store in the refrigerator until ready to eat.*

Nutritional information (per serving):
Calories: 382;
Protein: 11g;
Fat: 19g;
Carbohydrates: 43g;
Fiber: 7g

Turkey and Avocado Wrap

Servings: *1*

Ingredients:
1 whole wheat tortilla
2 oz. turkey breast
1/4 avocado, sliced
1/2 cup mixed greens
2 tbsp hummus
Salt and pepper to taste

Directions:
1. Lay the tortilla on a flat surface and spread hummus on top.
2. Add turkey breast, avocado slices, and mixed greens to the center of the tortilla.
3. Sprinkle with salt and pepper.
4. Fold the sides of the tortilla towards the center, then roll up tightly.
5. Cut the wrap in half and store in an airtight container until ready to eat.

Nutritional information (per serving):
Calories: 362;
Protein: 21g;
Fat: 18g;
Carbohydrates: 31g;
Fiber: 9g

Quinoa Salad with Roasted Vegetables

Servings: *4*

Ingredients:
1 cup quinoa
1 small sweet potato, peeled and diced
1 small red pepper, diced
1 small zucchini, diced
1 small yellow squash, diced
2 tbsp extra-virgin olive oil
1 tsp dried thyme
Salt and pepper to taste
1/4 cup crumbled feta cheese
2 tbsp lemon juice

Directions:
1. Preheat oven to 400°F.
2. In a large bowl, toss sweet potato, red pepper, zucchini, and yellow squash with olive oil, thyme, salt, and pepper.
3. Spread the vegetables in a single layer on a baking sheet and roast for 20-25 minutes, stirring occasionally, until tender.
4. Cook quinoa according to package directions until tender.
5. In a large bowl, combine cooked quinoa, roasted vegetables, feta cheese, and lemon juice.

6. Divide the quinoa salad into 4 containers and store in the refrigerator until ready to eat.

Nutritional information (per serving):
Calories: 312;
Protein: 9g;
Fat: 13g;
Carbohydrates: 43g;
Fiber: 7g

Southwest Quinoa Salad

Servings: *2*

Ingredients:
1 cup cooked quinoa
1/2 can black beans, drained and rinsed
1/2 cup corn kernels
1/2 red bell pepper, chopped
1/4 red onion, chopped
1/4 cup cilantro, chopped
Juice of 1 lime
Salt and pepper to taste

Directions:
1. In a large bowl, combine the quinoa, black beans, corn, red bell pepper, red onion, and cilantro.
2. Squeeze the lime juice over the mixture and toss to combine.
3. Season with salt and pepper to taste.
4. Divide the salad into two containers and refrigerate until ready to eat.

Nutritional information (per serving):
Calories: 310
Fat: 3.5g
Carbohydrates: 59g

Fiber: 12g
Protein: 14g

Chicken and Hummus Wrap

Servings: 1

Ingredients:
1 whole-wheat tortilla
2 tablespoons hummus
3 ounces grilled chicken breast, sliced
1/4 cup cucumber, sliced
1/4 cup cherry tomatoes, halved
1/4 cup lettuce, chopped

Directions:
1. Spread the hummus over the tortilla.
2. Add the sliced chicken, cucumber, cherry tomatoes, and lettuce on top of the hummus.
3. Roll the tortilla tightly and secure with a toothpick if necessary.
4. Pack the wrap in a container and refrigerate until ready to eat.

Nutritional information (per serving):
Calories: 340
Fat: 10g
Carbohydrates: 32g
Fiber: 8g
Protein: 34g

Veggie and Tuna Salad

Servings: *2*

Ingredients:
1 can tuna, drained

1/2 red bell pepper, chopped
1/2 cucumber, sliced
1/4 red onion, chopped
1/4 cup parsley, chopped
1 tablespoon olive oil
1 tablespoon lemon juice
Salt and pepper to taste
4 cups mixed greens

Directions:
1. In a large bowl, combine the tuna, red bell pepper, cucumber, red onion, parsley, olive oil, lemon juice, salt, and pepper.
2. Toss the ingredients together until the tuna is evenly coated.
3. Divide the mixed greens into two containers and top each with half of the tuna mixture.
4. Refrigerate until ready to eat.

Nutritional information (per serving):
Calories: 210
Fat: 10g
Carbohydrates: 9g
Fiber: 3g
Protein: 23g

Turkey and Cheese Wrap

Spread cream cheese on a whole wheat wrap, then add turkey, cheese, lettuce, and tomato.

Servings: *1*

Ingredients:
1 whole wheat wrap
2 tbsp cream cheese

2 slices deli turkey
1 slice cheddar cheese
1 leaf lettuce
2 slices tomato

Directions:
1. Spread the cream cheese on the wrap, then add the turkey, cheese, lettuce, and tomato.
2. Roll up tightly and slice in half.

Nutritional Information (per serving):
Calories: 310
Protein: 22g
Fat: 10g
Carbohydrates: 30g
Fiber: 7g
Sodium: 570mg

Asian Chicken Lettuce Wraps

Servings: *2*

Ingredients:
1 lb boneless, skinless chicken breasts, cut into small pieces
1 tablespoon vegetable oil
1/4 cup hoisin sauce
2 tablespoons soy sauce
2 tablespoons rice vinegar
1 tablespoon honey
1 garlic clove, minced
1/4 teaspoon red pepper flakes
8 large lettuce leaves
1/2 cup shredded carrots
1/4 cup sliced scallions

Directions:
1. Heat oil in a large skillet over medium-high heat.
2. Add chicken and cook until browned and cooked through, about 5-7 minutes.
3. In a small bowl, whisk together hoisin sauce, soy sauce, rice vinegar, honey, garlic, and red pepper flakes.
4. Add the sauce to the skillet and stir until chicken is evenly coated.
5. To serve, place a spoonful of chicken in each lettuce leaf, top with shredded carrots and scallions, and roll up tightly.

Nutritional Information (per serving):
Calories: 345
Fat: 10g
Carbohydrates: 28g
Protein: 38g
Fiber: 5g
Sodium: 1052mg

Greek Salad Pita

Servings: *2*

Ingredients:
2 whole wheat pita breads
2 tablespoons hummus
1/2 cup chopped cucumber
1/2 cup chopped cherry tomatoes
1/4 cup sliced red onion
1/4 cup sliced Kalamata olives
1/4 cup crumbled feta cheese
2 tablespoons Greek salad dressing

Directions:

1. Cut the pita breads in half and spread 1/2 tablespoon of hummus on each half.
2. Divide the cucumber, cherry tomatoes, red onion, Kalamata olives, and feta cheese between the pita halves.
3. Drizzle 1 tablespoon of Greek salad dressing over each pita half.
4. Fold each pita half in half and wrap in plastic wrap or aluminum foil to pack.

Nutritional Information (per serving):
Calories: 299
Fat: 13g
Carbohydrates: 37g
Protein: 10g
Fiber: 6g
Sodium: 741mg

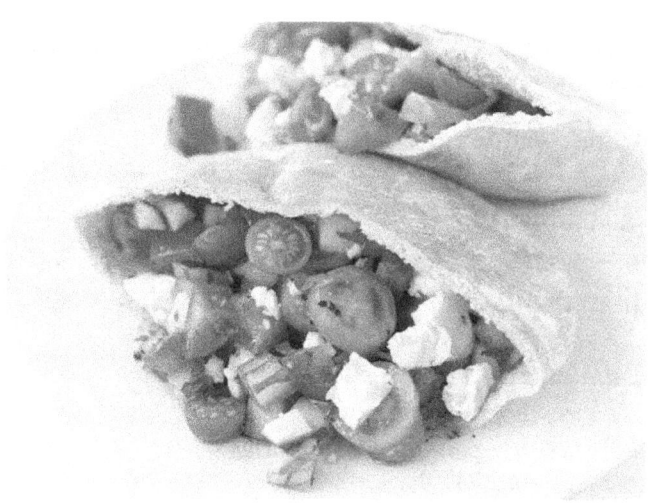

Panko-Crusted Cod

Panko are Japanese style breadcrumbs and provide a crunchy taste. Available in most supermarkets.

Servings: *2*

Ingredients:
1/4 Panko-style breadcrumbs
1 clove garlic, minced
1 tablespoon extra-virgin olive oil
3 tablespoons nonfat Greek yogurt
1 tablespoon mayonnaise
1 1/2 teaspoons lemon juice
1/2 teaspoon tarragon
Pinch of salt
10 ounces cod, cut into two portions

Directions:
1. Preheat oven to 425 degrees F. Coat baking pan with nonstick cooking spray.
2. In a small bowl, combine breadcrumbs, garlic and olive oil.
3. In another bowl, combine yogurt, mayonnaise, lemon juice, tarragon, and salt.
4. Place fish in baking pan. Top each piece with one half yogurt mixture and then 1/3 breadcrumb mixture.
5. Bake in oven for 15 minutes or until fish is opaque in center and breadcrumbs are golden brown.

Nutritional Information (per serving)
Calories: 225
Sodium: 270 mg
Protein: 18 g
Carbs: 13 g
Fat: 10 g

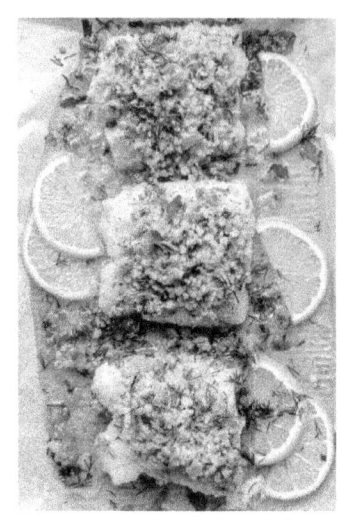

Steak Tacos

Authentic-style Mexican tacos.

Servings: *6*

Ingredients:
1 1/4 pounds sirloin steak, cut into strips
1/4 teaspoon salt
Freshly ground black pepper, to taste
2 tablespoons plus 2 teaspoons olive oil
12 (6-inch) tortillas
1/2 red onion, diced
3 fresh jalapeno peppers, seeded and chopped
1/2 bunch fresh cilantro, chopped
3 limes, cut into wedges

Directions:
1. In a large skillet, heat 2 tablespoons olive oil over medium-high heat. Add steak and sauté until browned on all sides and cooked through to desired

doneness, about 5-6 minutes. Season with salt and pepper. Remove from pan to plate and cover to keep warm.

2. In same skillet, add 2 more teaspoons olive oil and allow to get hot. Add tortillas, one at a time, and cook turning once, until tortilla is lightly browned but still flexible.

3. To assemble tacos, place tortilla on a plate and top with steak, onion, jalapeno peppers, and cilantro. Squeeze lime juice over top.

Nutritional Information (per serving)
Calories: 380
Sodium: 115 mg
Protein: 20 g
Carbs: 28 g
Fat: 21 g

Mediterranean Chickpea Salad

Servings: *2*

Ingredients:
1 can chickpeas, drained and rinsed
1 cucumber, chopped
1 red bell pepper, chopped
1/2 red onion, chopped
1/2 cup cherry tomatoes, halved
1/4 cup feta cheese, crumbled
2 tablespoons chopped fresh parsley
1 tablespoon chopped fresh dill
1/4 cup extra-virgin olive oil
1/4 cup fresh lemon juice
Salt and pepper to taste

Directions:

1. In a large bowl, combine chickpeas, cucumber, bell pepper, onion, tomatoes, feta, parsley, and dill.
2. In a small bowl, whisk together olive oil, lemon juice, salt, and pepper.
3. Pour the dressing over the chickpea mixture and toss to combine.
4. Divide the salad between two containers.

Nutritional Information (per serving):
Calories: 423
Protein: 13g
Fat: 26g
Carbs: 39g
Fiber: 12g
Sugar: 10g
Sodium: 558mg

Turkey and Hummus Wrap

Servings: *1*

Ingredients:
1 whole wheat tortilla
3 ounces sliced turkey breast
2 tablespoons hummus
1/2 cup baby spinach
1/4 cup sliced cucumber
1/4 cup sliced red bell pepper
Salt and pepper to taste

Directions:
1. Lay the tortilla flat on a cutting board.
2. Spread hummus on the tortilla.
3. Add turkey, spinach, cucumber, and red bell pepper to the center of the tortilla.
4. Sprinkle salt and pepper on top of the vegetables.

5. Fold in the sides of the tortilla, then roll it up from the bottom to create a wrap.
6. Place the wrap in a container.

Nutritional Information:
Calories: 349
Protein: 24g
Fat: 12g
Carbs: 38g
Fiber: 9g
Sugar: 5g
Sodium: 637mg

Quinoa Salad with Roasted Vegetables:

Servings: *2*

Ingredients:
1 cup cooked quinoa
1 red bell pepper, chopped
1 zucchini, chopped
1 red onion, chopped
1 tablespoon olive oil
Salt and pepper to taste
2 tablespoons chopped fresh parsley
2 tablespoons chopped fresh mint
1/4 cup crumbled feta cheese
2 tablespoons balsamic vinegar

Directions:
1. Preheat the oven to 425°F.
2. Toss the bell pepper, zucchini, and onion with olive oil, salt, and pepper. Spread the vegetables on a baking sheet.
3. Roast the vegetables for 20-25 minutes or until tender and lightly browned.

4. In a large bowl, combine cooked quinoa, roasted vegetables, parsley, mint, and feta cheese.
5. Drizzle balsamic vinegar over the salad and toss to combine.
6. Divide the salad between two containers.

Nutritional Information (per serving):
Calories: 369
Protein: 12g
Fat: 12g
Carbs: 57g
Fiber: 10g
Sugar: 12g
Sodium: 403mg

Turkey and Avocado Wrap

Servings: *2*

Ingredients:
2 whole wheat wraps
4 oz sliced turkey breast
1/2 avocado, sliced
1/2 cup baby spinach
2 tablespoons hummus

Directions:
1. Place the wraps on a flat surface.
2. Spread 1 tablespoon of hummus on each wrap.
3. Divide the sliced turkey, avocado, and baby spinach between the wraps.
4. Roll up tightly and wrap in plastic wrap or aluminum foil to pack

Nutritional Information (per serving):
Calories: 290

Fat: 13g
Carbohydrates: 27g
Protein: 17g
Fiber: 10g
Sodium: 575mg

Chickpea and Vegetable Salad

Servings: *2*

Ingredients:
1 can (15 oz) chickpeas, drained and rinsed
1/2 cup cherry tomatoes, halved
1/2 cup chopped cucumber
1/2 cup chopped bell pepper
1/4 cup chopped red onion
2 tablespoons chopped fresh parsley
2 tablespoons lemon juice
2 tablespoons olive oil
Salt and pepper to taste

Directions:
1. In a large bowl, combine the chickpeas, cherry tomatoes, cucumber, bell pepper, red onion, and parsley.
2. In a small bowl, whisk together the lemon juice, olive oil, salt, and pepper.
3. Drizzle the dressing over the salad and toss to combine.
4. Divide the salad between two containers and pack.

Nutritional Information (per serving):
Calories: 298
Fat: 14g
Carbohydrates: 34g

Protein: 11g
Fiber: 10g
Sodium: 295mg

Tuna Salad Lettuce Wraps

Servings: *2*

Ingredients:
1 can (5 oz) tuna, drained
1/4 cup diced celery
1/4 cup diced red onion
1 tablespoon chopped fresh dill
2 tablespoons lemon juice
1 tablespoon olive oil
Salt and pepper to taste
4 large lettuce leaves

Directions:
In a medium bowl, combine the tuna, celery, red onion, dill, lemon juice, olive oil, salt, and pepper.
Place 1/4 of the tuna salad mixture in the center of each lettuce leaf.
Roll up tightly and wrap in plastic wrap or aluminum foil to pack.

Nutritional Information (per serving):
Calories: 168
Fat: 8g
Carbohydrates: 5g
Protein: 19g
Fiber: 1g
Sodium: 314mg

Tuna Salad with Crackers

Servings: 1

Ingredients:
1 can of low-sodium tuna, drained
1 tablespoon plain Greek yogurt
1/2 tablespoon Dijon mustard
1/4 cup chopped celery
1/4 cup chopped red onion
6 whole-grain crackers
1/2 cup cherry tomatoes
1/2 cup baby carrots

Directions:
1. In a small bowl, mix together the tuna, Greek yogurt, Dijon mustard, celery, and red onion.
2. Pack the tuna salad and crackers in separate containers, along with cherry tomatoes and baby carrots on the side.

Nutritional Information:
Calories: 250
Protein: 23g
Fat: 7g
Carbohydrates: 25g
Fiber: 5g
Sodium: 400mg

Egg Salad with Veggie Wrap

Servings: 1

Ingredients:
2 hard-boiled eggs, chopped

1 tablespoon plain Greek yogurt
1/2 tablespoon Dijon mustard
1/4 cup chopped celery
1/4 cup chopped red onion
1 whole-grain tortilla
1/2 cup baby spinach leaves
1/4 cup shredded carrots
1/4 cup sliced cucumber

Directions:

1. In a small bowl, mix together the chopped hard-boiled eggs, Greek yogurt, Dijon mustard, celery, and red onion.

2. Place the whole-grain tortilla on a flat surface, and layer baby spinach leaves, shredded carrots, and sliced cucumber on top.

3. Spoon the egg salad over the veggies.

Roll up the tortilla tightly, tucking in the sides as you go.

4. Cut the wrap in half diagonally and pack in a lunchbox

.

Nutritional Information:

Calories: 320
Protein: 22g
Fat: 13g
Carbohydrates: 32g
Fiber: 9g
Sodium: 490mg

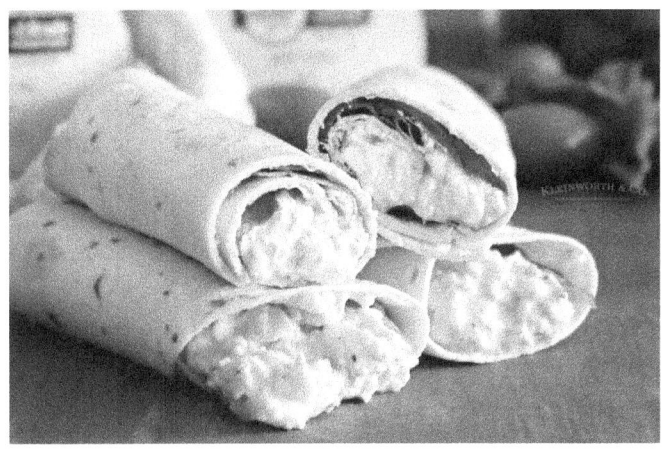

Sweet Potato Casserole

A crunchy pecan topping makes this feel like a decadent treat.

Servings: *8*

Ingredients:
2 1/4 cups sweet potatoes, peeled, cooked, and mashed
1/4 cup butter, melted
2 tablespoons low-fat milk
1/4 cup honey
1/4 teaspoon vanilla
1 egg, beaten
1/4 cup brown sugar
1/4 cup all-purpose flour
3 tablespoons butter
1/2 cup chopped pecans

Directions:
1. Preheat oven to 350 degrees F. Spray a 8 x 11 inch baking pan with cooking spray

2. In a large bowl, mix together sweet potatoes, melted butter, milk, honey, vanilla, and egg.
3. In a small bowl, mix together brown sugar and flour. Cut in 3 tablespoons butter until mixture is crumbly. Add pecans and stir.
4. Sprinkle pecan mixture over sweet potatoes.
5. Bank in oven for 25 minutes or until golden brown.

Nutritional Information (per serving)
Calories: 310
Sodium: 105 mg
Protein: 3.2 g
Carbs: 36 g
Fat: 13 g

Tips for meal prepping lunches for work

Meal prepping lunches for work can be a great way to save time, money, and ensure you're eating healthy throughout the workweek. With a little planning and preparation, you can have delicious, healthy meals ready to go, without the hassle of having to prepare meals every day. By following a few simple tips and tricks, you can create healthy, satisfying meals that will help you power through your workday. Whether you're looking to save time, eat healthier, or just simplify your life, meal prepping lunches for work is a great option. In this section, we'll share some tips and tricks for meal prepping lunches that are delicious, healthy, and easy to prepare.

1. **Plan your meals:** Spend some time planning your meals for the week. This will help you save time and avoid last-minute meal decisions.

2. **Batch cook:** Consider batch cooking on the weekends. Cook a large batch of protein, grains, and veggies, and then portion them out into containers for the week.

3. **Use your freezer:** Some meals freeze well, so take advantage of your freezer. Consider making large batches of soups, stews, and casseroles and freeze individual portions for later.

4. **Invest in good containers:** Invest in good quality food containers that are leak-proof and microwave-safe. Glass containers are a great option as they are safe for reheating and don't absorb odors.

5. **Keep it simple:** Choose meals that are simple to prepare and easy to transport. Salads, wraps, and sandwiches are all great options.

6. **Mix it up:** Don't get stuck in a rut with your meal prep. Mix up your meals and try new recipes to keep things interesting.

7. **Don't forget snacks:** Pack healthy snacks like fruit, nuts, and veggies to keep you satisfied between meals.

8. **Prep in advance:** Set aside a few hours on the weekend to prep your meals for the week. This will help you save time during the week and ensure you have healthy meals ready to go.

Easy lunch recipes that travel well

When you're on the go, finding healthy, satisfying meals can be a challenge. Whether you're running from meeting to meeting, traveling for work, or just trying to make it through a busy day, it's important to have meals that are easy to pack and travel well. Fortunately, there are plenty of easy lunch recipes that are not only delicious and nutritious, but also travel well. Whether you're looking for something that can be packed in a lunchbox, carried in a backpack, or enjoyed on the road, we've got you covered. In this section, we'll share some of our favorite easy lunch recipes that are perfect for busy professionals on the go. These recipes are simple to prepare, full of flavor, and designed to keep you fueled and satisfied throughout the day

Here are 10 easy lunch recipes that are perfect for busy professionals on the go. Each recipe is designed to be portable, easy to pack, and delicious.

Veggie wrap with hummus and avocado: Spread a tortilla with hummus, then add sliced avocado, cucumber, bell pepper, and lettuce. Roll up the tortilla tightly and cut in half.

Mason jar salad: Layer spinach, cherry tomatoes, shredded carrots, and quinoa in a mason jar. Add a dollop of pesto and a sprinkle of feta cheese on top. When ready to eat, shake the jar to mix everything together.

Greek yogurt parfait: Layer Greek yogurt, granola, and mixed berries in a jar or container. Drizzle with honey for added sweetness.

Peanut butter and banana sandwich: Spread peanut butter on two slices of whole grain bread. Add sliced banana and a drizzle of honey, then close the sandwich.

Chickpea salad: Mix canned chickpeas, diced cucumber, cherry tomatoes, and feta cheese in a bowl. Drizzle with olive oil and lemon juice, then pack in a container.

Chicken salad with crackers: Mix shredded chicken, diced celery, and dried cranberries in a bowl. Add a dollop of Greek yogurt and mix well. Pack with a handful of crackers.

Quinoa salad with roasted vegetables: Roast diced sweet potato, red onion, and bell pepper in the oven. Mix with cooked quinoa, spinach, and feta cheese. Drizzle with balsamic vinaigrette and pack in a container.

Tuna and bean salad: Mix canned tuna, canned white beans, diced red onion, and cherry tomatoes in a bowl. Add a drizzle of olive oil and red wine vinegar, then pack in a container.

Turkey and cheese roll-ups: Spread a tortilla with cream cheese, then add sliced turkey and cheese. Roll up the tortilla tightly and cut in half.

Apple and almond butter sandwich: Spread almond butter on two slices of whole grain bread.

Add sliced apple and a sprinkle of cinnamon, then close the sandwich.

These easy lunch recipes are perfect for busy professionals who are always on the go. With a little preparation, you can have delicious, healthy meals that travel well and keep you fueled throughout the day

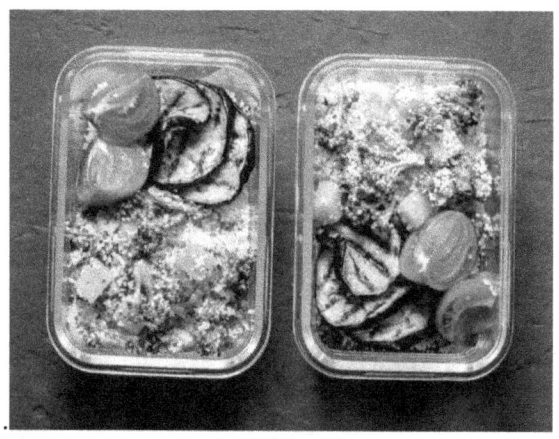

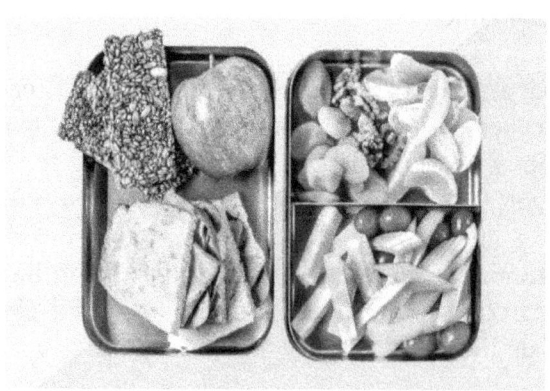

Chapter 4

Healthy Snacks to Fuel Your Day

Snacking is an essential part of maintaining a healthy and balanced diet, especially for busy professionals who often don't have time for a full meal. Snacks help to keep our energy levels up throughout the day and prevent us from overeating during our main meals. However, not all snacks are created equal, and unhealthy snack choices can quickly derail our healthy eating goals. That's why it's essential to have a collection of healthy snacks on hand that can help fuel your day and keep you feeling satisfied until your next meal. In this chapter, we'll explore some delicious and nutritious snack options that are easy to make, pack, and take with you on the go.

Ideas for portable snacks to keep you energized

Here are some ideas for portable snacks that can keep you energized throughout the day:

Trail mix: A mixture of nuts, seeds, dried fruit, and whole grain cereal is a great snack to keep in your bag. It's easy to make at home and is perfect for when you need a quick boost of energy.

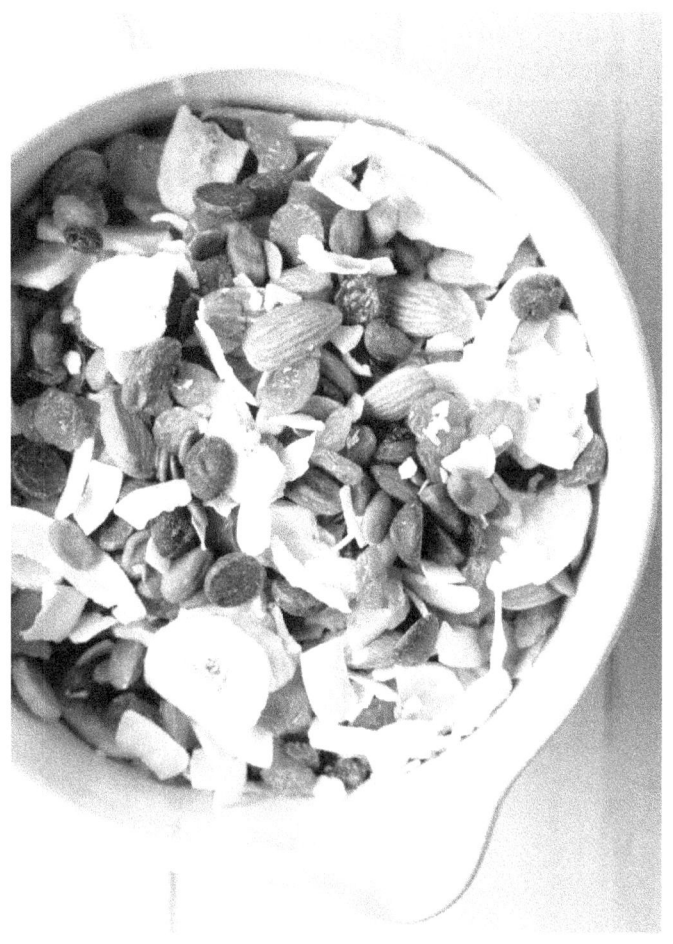

Fruit and nut butter: Apples, bananas, and carrots are excellent options to pair with nut butter. You can also try almond butter, cashew butter, or peanut butter for a delicious and filling snack.

Protein bars: Look for bars that are high in protein and low in added sugars. These bars are perfect for when you need a snack on the go, and they can help keep you full for hours.

Hummus and veggies: A cup of hummus with raw veggies such as carrots, celery, and cucumbers is a perfect combination of protein, fiber, and healthy fats.

Hard-boiled eggs: Hard-boiled eggs are an easy and portable snack that can keep you full for a long time. They're also rich in protein, healthy fats, and essential vitamins and minerals.

Greek yogurt: Greek yogurt is a great source of protein, and it can be paired with fresh fruit, granola, or nuts for a delicious and satisfying snack.

Energy balls: These homemade snacks are packed with nuts, seeds, dried fruit, and natural sweeteners like honey or maple syrup. They're easy to make and perfect for when you need a quick energy boost.

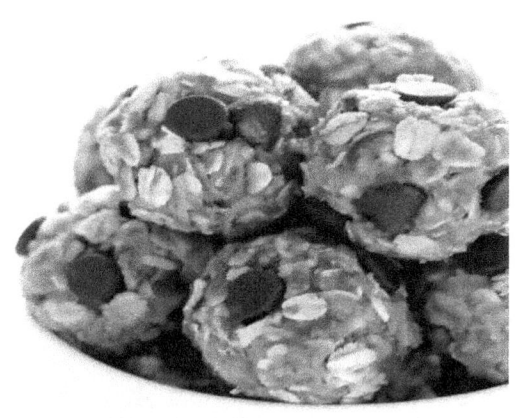

Cheese and whole grain crackers: Choose a low-fat cheese option and pair it with whole grain crackers for a snack that's high in protein and fiber.

Roasted chickpeas: Roasted chickpeas are a crunchy and flavorful snack that's also high in protein and fiber.

Smoothies: Smoothies made with fruit, vegetables, and protein powder are an excellent way to get a quick and nutritious snack when you're on the go. You can also make them ahead of time and take them with you in a portable container.

Simple recipes for quick and healthy snacks

Apple slices with almond butter

Servings: *1*

Ingredients:
1 medium apple, sliced
1 tablespoon almond butter

Directions:
1. Slice the apple into thin pieces.
2. Spread the almond butter over each slice.
Enjoy!

Nutritional information:
Calories: 179
Protein: 4g
Fat: 9g

Carbohydrates: 24g
Fiber: 5g

Greek yogurt with berries

Servings: *1*

Ingredients:
1/2 cup Greek yogurt
1/2 cup mixed berries (such as strawberries, blueberries, raspberries)

Directions:
1. Spoon the Greek yogurt into a bowl.
2. Top with the mixed berries.
Enjoy!

Nutritional information:
Calories: 120
Protein: 16g
Fat: 0g
Carbohydrates: 14g
Fiber: 2g

Carrots and hummus

Servings: *1*

Ingredients:
1 medium carrot, sliced
2 tablespoons hummus

Directions:
1. Slice the carrot into thin pieces.
2. Dip the carrot slices into the hummus.
Enjoy!

Nutritional information:
Calories: 90
Protein: 2g
Fat: 6g
Carbohydrates: 8g
Fiber: 3g

Trail mix

Servings: *1*

Ingredients:
1/4 cup almonds
1/4 cup cashews
1/4 cup dried cranberries
1/4 cup dark chocolate chips

Directions:
1. Mix all ingredients together in a small container.
Enjoy!

Nutritional information:
Calories: 326
Protein: 8g
Fat: 23g
Carbohydrates: 26g
Fiber: 3g

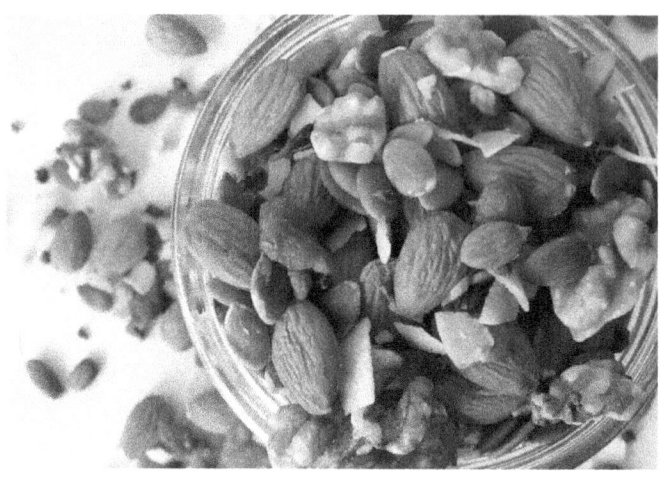

Roasted chickpeas

Servings: *2*

Ingredients:
1 can chickpeas, drained and rinsed
1 tablespoon olive oil
1/2 teaspoon salt
1/2 teaspoon garlic powder
1/2 teaspoon paprika

Directions:
1. Preheat the oven to 400°F (200°C).
2. In a bowl, mix together the chickpeas, olive oil, salt, garlic powder, and paprika.
3. Spread the mixture onto a baking sheet and bake for 20-25 minutes, or until golden brown and crispy.
4. Let cool before serving.

Nutritional information:
Calories: 224
Protein: 10g
Fat: 8g

Carbohydrates: 29g
Fiber: 9g

Peanut Butter and Apple Slices

Servings: *1*

Ingredients:
1 apple, sliced
2 tablespoons peanut butter

Directions:
1. Slice the apple into thin wedges.
2. Spread peanut butter on each apple slice.
3. Serve and enjoy!

Nutritional information:
Calories: 215
Fat: 16g
Carbohydrates: 17g
Protein: 7g

Cottage Cheese and Pineapple

Servings: *1*

Ingredients:
1/2 cup cottage cheese
1/2 cup fresh pineapple chunks

Directions:
1. Spoon the cottage cheese into a small container.
2. Add the fresh pineapple chunks on top of the cottage cheese.
3. Cover and refrigerate until ready to eat.

Nutritional information:
Calories: 110
Fat: 1g
Carbohydrates: 16g
Protein: 11g

Energy Balls

Servings: *10-12 balls*

Ingredients:
1 cup rolled oats
1/2 cup almond butter
1/4 cup honey
1/4 cup ground flaxseed
1/4 cup mini chocolate chips
1 tsp vanilla extract

Directions:
1. In a mixing bowl, combine all ingredients until well combined.
2. Cover the mixture and chill in the refrigerator for at least 30 minutes.
3. Using a cookie scoop or spoon, form the mixture into balls.
4. Store in an airtight container in the refrigerator for up to a week.

Nutritional Information (per serving):
Calories: 165
Protein: 4g
Fat: 9g
Carbohydrates: 20g
Fiber: 3g
Sugar: 10g

Hummus and Veggies

Servings: *2*

Ingredients:
1/2 cup hummus
2 carrots, sliced
1 red bell pepper, sliced
1/2 cucumber, sliced

Directions:
1. Divide the hummus into two containers with lids.
2. Add the sliced veggies to each container.
3. Seal the containers and refrigerate until ready to eat.

Nutritional Information (per serving):
Calories: 170
Protein: 5g
Fat: 9g
Carbohydrates: 19g
Fiber: 7g
Sugar: 6g

Cheese and Whole Grain Crackers

Servings: *1*

Ingredients:
1 oz cheddar cheese
5 whole grain crackers

Directions:
1. Pack the cheese and crackers in a small container or plastic bag.

2. Refrigerate until ready to eat.

Nutritional Information (per serving):
Calories: 160
Protein: 8g
Fat: 9g
Carbohydrates: 14g
Fiber: 2g
Sugar: 1g

Carrot Cake Cookies

These cookies are full of carrot cake flavor in every bit.

Servings: *24 cookies*

Ingredients
1/4 cup packed light-brown sugar
1/4 cup sugar
1/4 cup oil
1/4 cup applesauce or fruit puree
1 eggs
1/2 teaspoon vanilla
1/2 cup flour
1/2 cup whole wheat flour
1/2 teaspoon baking soda
1/2 teaspoon baking powder
1/8 teaspoon salt
1/2 teaspoon ground cinnamon
1/4 teaspoon ground nutmeg
1/4 teaspoon ground ginger
1 cups old-fashioned rolled oats (raw)
3/4 cup finely grated carrots (about 2 carrots)
1/2 cup raisins or golden raisins

Directions:
1. Preheat oven to 350 degrees F.
2. Mix together sugars, oil, applesauce, egg, and vanilla.
3. In a separate bowl, mix together all dry ingredients.
4. Add dry ingredients into wet ingredients. Mix until just blended. Stir in
carrots and raisins.
5. Drop by teaspoonful on parchment-lined cookie sheet.
6. Bake 12-14 minutes or until golden brown.

Nutritional Information (per cookie)
Calories: 80
Sodium: 55 mg
Protein: 1 g
Carbs: 13 g
Fat: 3 g

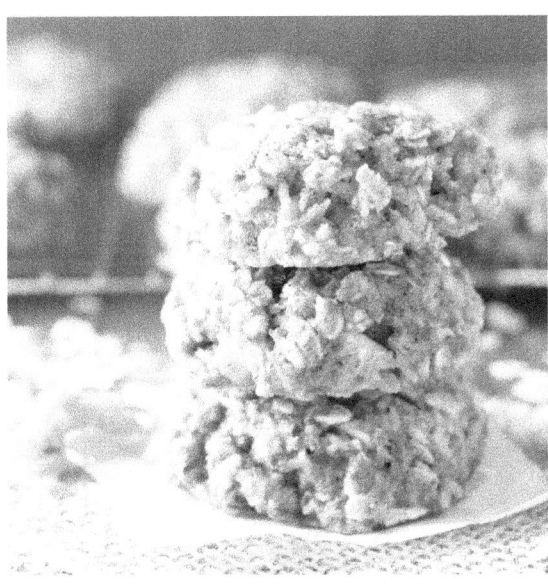

Microwave-Baked Stuffed Apples

Perfect for dessert on a crisp autumn day.

Servings: *4*

Ingredients:
4 large apples
1/4 cup coconut flakes
1/4 cup dried cranberries or apricots
2 teaspoons orange zest, grated
1/2 cup orange juice
2 tablespoons brown sugar

Directions:
1. Cut top off apple and hollow out center with knife or apple corer. Arrange apples in a microwave-safe dish.
2. In a bowl, combine coconut, cranberries, and orange zest. Divide evenly and fill centers of apples.
3. In a bowl, mix orange juice and brown sugar. Pour over apples. Cover with microwave-safe plastic wrap and microwave on high for 7-8 minutes or until apples are tender.
3. Serve warm.

Nutritional Information (per serving)
Calories: 190
Sodium: 275 mg
Protein: 1 g
Carbs: 46 g
Fat: 2 g

Oatmeal Walnut Chocolate Chip Cookies

We've reduced the amount of saturated fat in these cookies without sacrificing any of the taste.

Servings: 24 cookies

Ingredients:
1 cup rolled oats (not quick-cooking)
1/4 cup all-purpose flour
1/4 cup whole-wheat pastry flour
1/2 teaspoon ground cinnamon
1/4 teaspoon baking soda
1/4 teaspoon salt
1/4 cup tahini (sesame seed paste)
4 tablespoons cold unsalted butter, cut into pieces
1/3 cup granulated sugar
1/3 cup packed light brown sugar
1 large egg
1/2 tablespoon vanilla extract
1/2 cup semisweet or bittersweet chocolate chips
1/4 cup chopped walnuts

Directions:
1. Preheat oven to 350 degrees F. Line 2 cookie sheets with parchment paper.
2. Mix together oats, flour, cinnamon, baking soda, and salt in bowl.
3. In another large bowl, whisk together tahini, butter, sugar, brown sugar, egg, and vanilla until smooth.
4. Add in oat mixture and mix until just moistened.
5. Stir in chocolate chips and walnuts.

6. *Place tablespoon-size portions of batter on cookie sheets, allowing space between.*
7. *Bake for about 14-16 minutes or until cookies are golden brown.*

Note: Tahini can be substituted with almond butter or other nut butter.

Nutritional Information (per cookie)
Calories: 110
Sodium: 45 mg
Protein: 2 g
Carbs: 15 g
Fat: 5 g

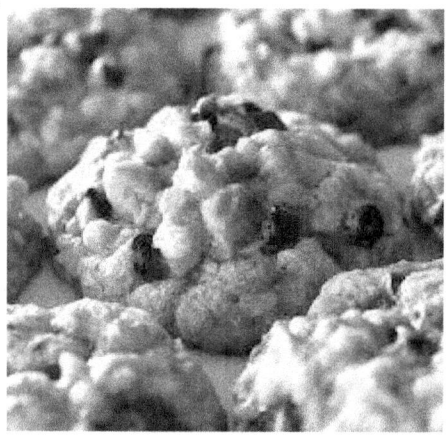

Chapter 5

Quick and Easy Dinner Ideas

In today's fast-paced world, finding time to prepare a healthy and satisfying dinner can be a challenge, especially for busy professionals. However, with the right strategies and recipes, it is possible to create quick and easy dinners that are not only delicious but also nutritious. This chapter is dedicated to providing you with a collection of dinner ideas that are simple, healthy, and can be prepared in 30 minutes or less. From vegetarian options to meat-based dishes, these recipes are designed to help you eat well, even on the busiest of days.

One-pot meals for a quick and healthy dinner

One-pot meals are a great solution for those who want to create a healthy and satisfying dinner with minimal effort and cleanup. These meals are easy to prepare, and all you need is one pot or pan to make them. In this section, we will explore a variety of one-pot meal ideas that are quick, healthy, and delicious. Whether you're looking for vegetarian options or want to incorporate some protein into your meal, these recipes are sure to become a staple in your dinner rotation. With the convenience of one-pot meals, you can spend less time in the kitchen and more time enjoying your meal and relaxing after a long day.

One-Pot Chicken and Rice

Servings: *4*

Ingredients:
1 pound boneless, skinless chicken breasts, cut into bite-sized pieces
1 tablespoon olive oil
1 onion, diced
1 red bell pepper, diced
2 cloves garlic, minced
1 teaspoon dried thyme
1/2 teaspoon smoked paprika
1 cup brown rice
2 cups chicken broth
1 (15-ounce) can black beans, drained and rinsed
Salt and pepper to taste

Directions:
1. In a large pot or Dutch oven, heat the olive oil over medium-high heat. Add the chicken and cook until browned on all sides, about 5-7 minutes.
2. Remove the chicken from the pot and set aside.
3. Add the onion, red bell pepper, and garlic to the pot and sauté for 2-3 minutes, until slightly softened. Add the thyme and smoked paprika and cook for 1-2 minutes, until fragrant.
4. Add the rice and chicken broth to the pot and stir to combine. Bring the mixture to a boil, then reduce the heat to low and cover the pot with a lid. Simmer for 25-30 minutes, until the rice is tender and the liquid is absorbed.
5. Add the cooked chicken and black beans to the pot and stir to combine. Season with salt and pepper to taste. Serve hot.

Nutritional information per serving:
Calories: 418
Fat: 8g
Carbohydrates: 53g
Protein: 32g
Sodium: 650 mg

One-Pot Vegetable Pasta

Servings: *4*

Ingredients:
8 ounces whole wheat pasta
1 tablespoon olive oil
1 onion, diced
2 cloves garlic, minced
2 carrots, peeled and sliced
2 cups sliced mushrooms
1 red bell pepper, diced
1 zucchini, diced
1 (14-ounce) can diced tomatoes
2 cups vegetable broth
Salt and pepper to taste

Directions:
1. In a large pot or Dutch oven, heat the olive oil over medium-high heat. Add the onion and garlic and sauté for 2-3 minutes, until slightly softened.
2. Add the carrots, mushrooms, red bell pepper, and zucchini to the pot and sauté for 5-7 minutes, until the vegetables are slightly tender.
3. Add the diced tomatoes, vegetable broth, and pasta to the pot and stir to combine. Bring the mixture to a boil, then reduce the heat to low and cover the pot with a lid. Simmer for 10-12 minutes, until the pasta is tender and the liquid is absorbed.

4. Season with salt and pepper to taste. Serve hot.

Nutritional information per serving:
Calories: 286
Fat: 5g
Carbohydrates: 52g
Protein: 13g
Sodium: 415 mg

Whole-Wheat Spaghetti with Ragu Sauce

Store-bought spaghetti sauce is full of sodium. Try this easy, homemade version instead for a healthy meal.

Servings: *8*

Ingredients:
1 box whole-wheat spaghetti
1 tablespoon extra-virgin olive oil
1 medium onion, chopped fine
1 large carrot, chopped fine
1 stalk celery, chopped fine
4 cloves garlic, minced
1 teaspoon oregano
1 teaspoon basil
1 teaspoon marjoram
1 pound lean ground beef
1 28-ounce can crushed tomatoes, no salt added
1/2 teaspoon salt
1/4 cup flat-leaf parsley, chopped
1/2 cup grated Parmesan cheese

Directions:

1. *Cook spaghetti according to package directions. Drain.*
2. *While pasta cooks, heat oil in large skillet over medium heat. Add onion, carrot, and celery and cooking, stirring occasionally, until onion turns translucent, about 5 minutes. Add in garlic and seasonings, and cook for another 30 seconds.*
3. *Add beef and cook, stirring, until meat is browned and no longer pink,*
about 4-5 minutes. Add crushed tomatoes and continue to cook, stirring occasionally, until sauce thickens, about 5 minutes. Season with salt and add parsley.
4. *To serve, plate 1 cup of pasta, top with sauce and sprinkle with Parmesan cheese.*

Note: Sauce can be made ahead and kept in the refrigerator for up to 3 days.

Nutritional Information (per serving):
Calories: 385
Sodium: 415 mg
Protein: 28 g
Carbs: 52 g
Fat: 9 g

Grilled Salmon and Asparagus with Lemon Butter

Salmon is rich in heart-healthy omega-3s. Buy wild salmon whenever possible.

Servings: *4*

Ingredients:
1 1/4 pounds salmon, cut into 4 portions

2 bunches asparagus, ends trimmed
Cooking spray, preferably olive oil
1/2 teaspoon salt
1/4 teaspoon freshly ground pepper
1/4 teaspoon garlic powder
1 tablespoon olive oil
1 tablespoon butter
3 tablespoons lemon juice

Directions:

1. Place salmon and asparagus on large rimmed baking sheet. Spray lightly with cooking spray. Sprinkle with salt, pepper, and garlic powder.
2. Place asparagus and salmon on preheated, oiled grill. Grill the salmon, turning once, until opaque, about 3-5 minutes per side. Grill the asparagus, turning occasionally, until tender, about 5-7 minutes.
5. In a microwave-safe bowl, place olive oil, butter, and lemon juice. Microwave to melt butter, about 20 seconds. Drizzle fish with butterlemon mixture. Serve immediately.

Note: This can also be cooked under the broiler instead of the grill.

Nutritional Information (per serving):

Calories: 190
Sodium: 445 mg
Protein: 24 g
Carbs: 6 g
Fat: 8 g

Steak Smothered in Mushrooms

Sirloin steak topped with mushrooms in a balsamic sauce.

Servings: *4*

Ingredients:
1 pound sirloin steak
1 tablespoon olive oil
1 1/2 cups mushrooms, sliced
2 tablespoons butter
1/2 tablespoon all-purpose flour
Freshly ground black pepper, to taste
3 tablespoons balsamic vinegar

Directions:
1. Heat oil in large nonstick skillet over medium-high heat. Add steak and cook, turning once, until desired doneness. Remove steak from pan and slice into thin strips.
2. In same skillet, add mushrooms and butter. Sprinkle with flour and continue cooking, stirring occasionally, until mushrooms start to brown. About 5-6 minutes. Season with black pepper.
3. Add in vinegar and cook for an additional 2 minutes, stirring frequently.
4. Serve steak with mushroom mixture on top.

Nutritional Information (per serving):
Calories: 175
Sodium: 105 mg
Protein: 30 g
Carbs: 8 g
Fat: 2 g

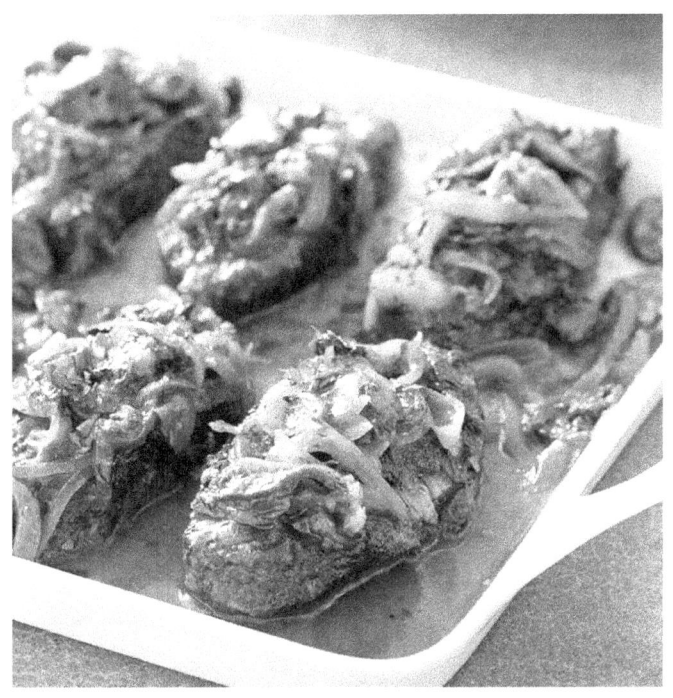

Mediterranean Lemon Chicken and Potatoes

Servings: *4*

Ingredients:
*1 1/2 pounds chicken breast, skinless and boneless,
cut into 1-inch cubes*
1 pound Yukon Gold potatoes, cut into cubes
1 medium onion, chopped
1 red or yellow pepper, chopped
1/2 cup low-sodium vinaigrette
1/4 cup lemon juice
1 teaspoon oregano
1/2 teaspoon garlic powder
1/2 cup chopped tomato

Freshly ground black pepper, to taste

Directions:
1. Mix all ingredients except tomatoes together in large bowl.
2. Lay out 4 large squares of aluminum foil. Place equal amount of chicken and potato mixture in the center of each square. Fold top and sides to enclose mixture in packet.
3. Bake in preheated 400 degree F oven for 30 minutes or until chicken and potatoes are cooked through. Packet may also be cooked on the grill.
4. Open packets and top with chopped tomatoes. Season with black pepper to taste.

Nutritional Information (per serving)
Calories: 320
Sodium: 420 mg
Protein: 43 g
Carbs: 34 g
Fat: 4 g

Lemon Garlic Shrimp and Broccoli Quinoa

Servings: *4*

Ingredients:
1 pound large shrimp, peeled and deveined
1 head broccoli, chopped
1 cup uncooked quinoa
2 cups low-sodium chicken broth
2 cloves garlic, minced
1 lemon, juiced and zested
1 tablespoon olive oil
Salt and pepper to taste

Directions:

1. Heat olive oil in a large pot over medium heat.
2. Add garlic and cook until fragrant, about 30 seconds.
3. Add quinoa, chicken broth, lemon juice, and lemon zest to the pot and stir to combine.
4. Bring mixture to a boil, then reduce heat to low and cover the pot.
5. Cook for 15-20 minutes or until quinoa is tender. Add broccoli and shrimp to the pot and cook for an additional 5-7 minutes or until shrimp is pink and cooked through.
6. Season with salt and pepper to taste.

Nutrition information per serving:

Calories: 335
Protein: 32g
Fat: 7g
Carbohydrates: 37g
Fiber: 6g
Sodium: 384mg

Chicken Fajita Pasta

Servings: 4

Ingredients:

1 pound boneless, skinless chicken breast, cut into bite-sized pieces
1 green bell pepper, sliced
1 red bell pepper, sliced
1 yellow onion, sliced
2 cloves garlic, minced
2 cups low-sodium chicken broth
2 cups uncooked whole wheat pasta

Directions:
1. Heat olive oil in a large pot over medium heat.
2. Add chicken breast into the pot and cook until browned on all sides, about 5-7 minutes.
3. Add bell peppers, onion, and garlic to the pot and cook for an additional 3-4 minutes or until vegetables are tender.
4. Add chicken broth, uncooked pasta, chili powder, cumin, salt, and pepper to the pot and stir to combine.
5. Bring mixture to a boil, then reduce heat to low and cover the pot. Cook for 15-20 minutes or until pasta is tender and most of the liquid has been absorbed. Serve hot.

Nutrition information per serving:
Calories: 383
Protein: 34g
Fat: 7g
Carbohydrates: 46g
Fiber: 7g
Sodium: 309mg

Sweet Potato and Black Bean Chili

Servings: *6*

Ingredients:
2 large sweet potatoes, peeled and chopped
1 yellow onion, diced
1 red bell pepper, diced
1 green bell pepper, diced
2 cloves garlic, minced
1 can (15 ounces) black beans, drained and rinsed

1 can (28 ounces) diced tomatoes
2 cups low-sodium vegetable broth
2 teaspoons chili powder
1 teaspoon cumin
Salt and pepper to taste
1 tablespoon olive oil

Directions:

1. Heat olive oil in a large pot over medium heat.

2. Add onion and garlic to the pot and cook until softened, about 3-4 minutes.

3. Add sweet potatoes and bell peppers to the pot and cook for an additional 5-7 minutes or until vegetables are slightly tender.

4. Add black beans, diced tomatoes, vegetable broth, chili powder, cumin, salt, and pepper to the pot and stir to combine.

5. Bring mixture to a boil, then reduce heat to low and cover the pot.

Cook for 20-25 minutes or until sweet potatoes are tender. Serve hot.

Nutrition information per serving:

Calories: 220
Protein: 8g
Fat: 3g
Carbohydrates: 44g
Fiber: 10g
Sodium: 260mg

Vegetable Fried Rice

Servings: *4*

Ingredients:

2 cups cooked brown rice
2 tablespoons low-sodium soy sauce
1 tablespoon sesame oil
1 tablespoon olive oil
1 onion, diced
1 cup frozen mixed vegetables
2 cloves garlic, minced
2 eggs, beaten
Salt and pepper to taste

Directions:
1. Heat olive oil in a large skillet over medium heat.
2. Add onion and garlic to the skillet and cook until softened, about 3-4 minutes.
3. Add frozen mixed vegetables to the skillet and cook for an additional 3-4 minutes or until vegetables are slightly tender.
4. Push vegetables to the side of the skillet and add beaten eggs to the other side.
5. Scramble the eggs until cooked through, then mix with the vegetables.
6. Add cooked brown rice, soy sauce, sesame oil, salt, and pepper to the skillet and stir to combine. Cook for an additional 2-3 minutes or until everything is heated through. Serve hot.

Nutrition information per serving:
Calories: 296
Protein: 11g
Fat: 10g
Carbohydrates: 42g
Fiber: 6g
Sodium: 451mg

Lemon Garlic Shrimp and Broccoli Skillet

Servings: *4*

Ingredients:
1 pound large shrimp, peeled and deveined
1 tablespoon olive oil
1 tablespoon butter
1/2 onion, chopped
3 cloves garlic, minced
1 broccoli crown, chopped
1 lemon, juiced and zested
Salt and pepper, to taste

Directions:
1. Heat the olive oil and butter in a large skillet over medium heat.
2. Add the onion and garlic and cook until the onion is translucent, about 5 minutes.
3. Add the shrimp and cook until pink, about 2-3 minutes per side.
4. Add the chopped broccoli and lemon juice and cook for an additional 3-4 minutes, until the broccoli is tender-crisp.
5. Season with salt and pepper to taste. Serve hot.

Nutritional Information per serving:
Calories: 187
Fat: 8g
Carbohydrates: 9g
Fiber: 3g
Protein: 21g
Sodium: 325mg

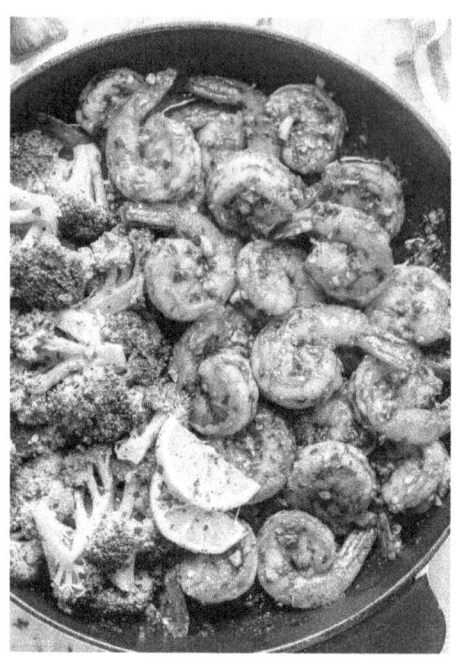

Quinoa and Black Bean Skillet

Servings: *4*

Ingredients:
1 tablespoon olive oil
1/2 onion, chopped
3 cloves garlic, minced
1 red bell pepper, chopped
1 can black beans, drained and rinsed
1 can diced tomatoes
1 cup quinoa, rinsed
2 cups vegetable broth
Salt and pepper, to taste
Cilantro, chopped, for garnish

Directions:

1. Heat the olive oil in a large skillet over medium heat.
2. Add the onion and garlic and cook until the onion is translucent, about 5 minutes.
3. Add the red bell pepper and cook for an additional 3-4 minutes.
4. Add the black beans, diced tomatoes, quinoa, and vegetable broth to the skillet and bring to a boil.
5. Reduce the heat to low, cover, and simmer for 15-20 minutes, until the quinoa is tender. Season with salt and pepper to taste.
6. Serve hot, garnished with cilantro.

Nutritional Information per serving:
Calories: 330
Fat: 6g
Carbohydrates: 58g
Fiber: 15g
Protein: 14g
Sodium: 559mg

Beef and Vegetable Stir-Fry

Servings: *4*

Ingredients:
1 pound beef sirloin, sliced
2 tablespoons soy sauce
2 tablespoons hoisin sauce
1 tablespoon cornstarch
1 tablespoon olive oil
1/2 onion, sliced
1 red bell pepper, sliced
2 cups broccoli florets
2 cloves garlic, minced
Salt and pepper, to taste

Directions:
1. In a small bowl, whisk together the soy sauce, hoisin sauce, and cornstarch.
2. Heat the olive oil in a large skillet or wok over high heat.
3. Add the beef and cook until browned, about 3-4 minutes.
4. Add the onion, red bell pepper, broccoli, and garlic to the skillet and cook for an additional 3-4 minutes, until the vegetables are tender-crisp. Pour the sauce over the beef and vegetables and stir to combine.
5. Cook for an additional 1-2 minutes, until the sauce has thickened.
6. Season with salt and pepper to taste. Serve hot.

Orange Chicken and Broccoli Stir Fry

Skip the Chinese takeout and serve this delicious healthy stir fry instead.

Servings: *4*

Ingredients:
1 tablespoon olive oil or coconut oil
1 pound chicken breast, boneless and skinless, cut into strips
1/3 cup orange juice
2 tablespoons low-sodium soy sauce
2 teaspoons cornstarch
2 cups broccoli, cut into small pieces
1 cup snow peas
2 cups cabbage, shredded
2 cups brown rice, cooked

1 tablespoon sesame seeds (optional)

Directions:
1. In a bowl, combine orange juice, soy sauce, and corn starch. Set aside.
2. Heat oil in wok or large sauté pan. Add chicken and stir fry for 4-5 minutes or until chicken is golden brown on all sides.
3. Add broccoli, snow peas, cabbage, and sauce mixture. Continue to stir fry until vegetables are tender but still crisp, about 7-8 minutes.
4. Serve over brown rice and sprinkle with sesame seeds.

Nutritional Information (per serving)
Calories: 340
Sodium: 240 mg
Protein: 28 g
Carbs: 35 g
Fat: 8g

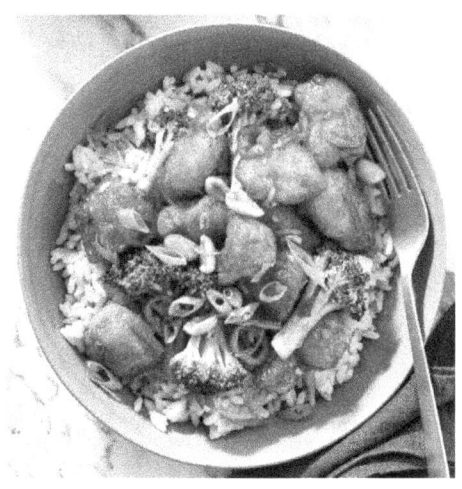

Simple Baked Chicken

This is a simple, classic dish.

Servings: *4*

Ingredients:
· *3-4 pound chicken, cut into parts*
· *2-3 tablespoons olive oil*
· *1/2 teaspoon thyme*
· *1/4 teaspoon sea salt*
· *Freshly ground black pepper*
· *1/2 cup low-sodium chicken stock*

Directions:
1. Preheat oven to 400 degrees F.
2. Trim off any excess fat from chicken pieces. Rinse and pat dry with paper towels.
3. Rub olive oil over chicken pieces. Sprinkle with thyme, salt, and pepper.
4. Arrange chicken pieces in roasting pan.
5. Bake chicken in oven for 30 minutes. Lower heat to 350 degrees F and bake for an addition 15-30 minutes, or until juice run clear.
6. Remove from oven. Let rest for 5 to 10 minutes before serving.

Nutritional Information (per serving)
Calories: 550
Sodium: 480 mg
Protein: 91 g
Carbs: 0 g
Fat: 19 g

Chicken Alfredo with Whole-Wheat Bowtie *Pasta*

Servings: *6*

Ingredients:
12 ounces whole wheat bowtie pasta
2 tablespoons olive oil
3 chicken breasts, boneless and skinless
2 cloves garlic
3/4 low-sodium chicken broth
1/2 cup half-and-half
3/4 cup grated Parmesan cheese
2 tablespoons fresh parsley, minced
Freshly ground black pepper, to taste

Directions:
1. Cook pasta according to package directions. Drain and set aside.
2. In a large skillet, heat 2 tablespoons of olive oil over medium-high heat. Add chicken breasts and cook until golden brown and done in the middle, about 5-6 minutes per side. Remove from pan, slice into bite-size pieces, set aside.
3. Add remaining 2 tablespoons of olive oil to pan. Add garlic and sauté for 1 minute. Pour in broth and let it boil for about 2 minutes. Add half-and-half and whisk together. Continuing cooking, stirring frequently, for several minutes until liquid starts to thicken.
4. Remove pan from and add Parmesan cheese, chicken, and pasta. Season with black pepper. Toss all ingredients together until well combined. If

sauce is too thick, add a little extra chicken broth to thin it down.

5. Serve topped with parsley and additional Parmesan cheese, if desired.

Nutritional Information (per serving)
Calories: 490
Sodium: 450 mg
Protein: 28 g
Carbs: 46 g
Fat: 19 g

Quick and Easy Chili

Great-tasting, this chili can be prepared with just a few ingredients.

Servings: *6*
Ingredients:
1/2 pound lean ground beef
1/2 medium yellow onion, diced
1 can (15.5) low-sodium kidney beans, drained
1 can (14.5 ounces) diced tomatoes
1 1/2 tablespoons chili powder

Directions:
1. In a large skillet brown ground meat and onions over medium-high heat (about 6-7 minutes). Drain excess fat.
2. Add beans, tomatoes, and chili powder.
3. Reduce heat to low, cover, and simmer for 10 minutes.
4. Serve with brown rice.

Nutritional Information (per serving)
Calories: 220

Sodium: 430 mg
Protein: 16 g
Carbs: 21 g
Fat: 7 g

Pasta Primavera with Shrimp and Spinach *Fettuccine*

Packed with veggies, this meal is tasty and quick.

Servings: *6*

Ingredients:
1/2 pound fresh asparagus, trimmed, cut into 1-inch lengths
12 ounces spinach fettuccine (can substitute whole-wheat if desired)
2 teaspoons olive oil
3 garlic cloves, minced
1/4 teaspoon crushed red pepper
1 pound medium shrimp, peeled and deveined (thawed if frozen)
1 cup green peas, fresh or frozen
1/2 cup green onion, sliced thin
1 tablespoon lemon juice
1 tablespoon fresh parsley, chopped
1/3 cup Parmesan cheese, grated
1/2 teaspoon salt
Freshly ground black pepper, to taste

Directions:
1. Fill a large pot with water and bring to a boil. Add asparagus and cook until tender but still crisp, about 4 minutes. Remove from water with slotted spoon and set aside. Add pasta to water and cooking according to package directions. Set aside.

2. In a large skillet, heat olive oil over medium heat. Add garlic and crushed red pepper and cook, stirring, for about a minute. Add shrimp, peas, and green onion and cook, stirring, for 3-4 minutes.
3. Add reserved pasta and asparagus along with lemon juice, parsley, and Parmesan cheese. Season with salt and pepper. Toss to coat.
4. Serve hot.

Nutritional Information (per serving)
Calories: 360
Sodium: 380 mg
Protein: 26 g
Carbs: 49 g
Fat: 6 g

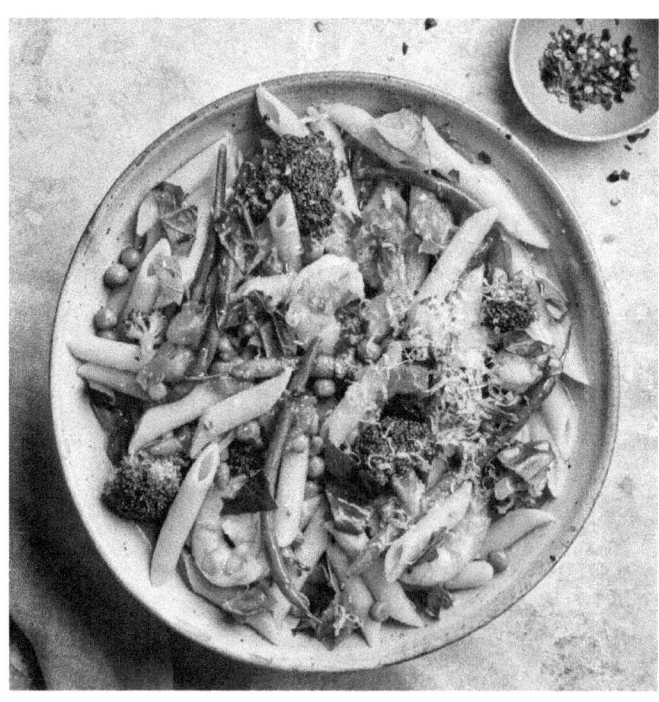

Meal planning and prepping is an excellent way to save time and make sure you have healthy meals available throughout the week. Here are some tips to help you get started:

Plan your meals for the week: Start by creating a meal plan for the week, taking into consideration your schedule and the foods you have on hand. You can use a planner, a notebook or an app to keep track of your meal plans.

Make a grocery list: Once you have your meal plan in place, create a grocery list of all the ingredients you will need for the week. This will help you avoid multiple trips to the store.

Prep ingredients in advance: You can save time by prepping some ingredients in advance. For example, you can chop vegetables, cook rice, or marinate meat the night before.

Cook in bulk: Cooking in bulk can save time and ensure you have leftovers for the next day. You can cook a big pot of soup, chili, or stew and portion it out for the week.

Use time-saving appliances: Appliances like slow cookers, instant pots, or air fryers can save you time in the kitchen. You can set them up in the morning and come home to a hot meal.

Freeze meals for later: You can also cook extra meals and freeze them for later. This is especially helpful for busy nights when you don't have time to cook.

By following these tips, you can streamline your meal planning and prep, making it easier to eat healthy, delicious meals throughout the week.

Chapter 6

DASH Diet Desserts

Maintaining a healthy and balanced diet doesn't mean you have to give up desserts entirely. It's a common misconception that indulging in sweets is off-limits when following a healthy diet. In reality, there are many ways to satisfy your sweet tooth without sabotaging your health goals. With the DASH diet, you can still enjoy sweet treats in moderation. The key is to choose ingredients that are rich in nutrients and low in added sugars. In this chapter, we will explore some delicious and easy-to-make DASH diet desserts that will satisfy your sweet tooth while keeping you on track with your health goals. From fruity delights to chocolatey indulgences, there's something for everyone to enjoy. So, let's dive in and discover some tasty DASH diet desserts

Healthy dessert ideas that won't compromise your diet

Berry Chia Seed Pudding

Servings: *2*

Ingredients:
1/4 cup chia seeds
1 cup unsweetened almond milk
1/2 tsp vanilla extract

1 tbsp honey
1/2 cup mixed berries

Directions:
1. In a mixing bowl, whisk together chia seeds, almond milk, vanilla extract, and honey.
2. Let the mixture sit for 5 minutes and then whisk again.
3. Cover the bowl and refrigerate overnight. Top with mixed berries before serving.

Nutritional Information (per serving):
Calories: 205
Fat: 9.3g
Carbohydrates: 27.8g
Fiber: 11g
Protein: 5.6g
Sodium: 88mg

Baked Apples

Servings: 2

Ingredients:
2 apples, cored and sliced
1 tsp cinnamon
1/4 tsp nutmeg
1 tbsp honey
1/4 cup chopped walnuts

Directions:
1. Preheat oven to 375°F.
2. In a mixing bowl, toss apples with cinnamon, nutmeg, and honey.
3. Place the apples in a baking dish and sprinkle with chopped walnuts.

4. Bake for 20-25 minutes or until the apples are tender.

Nutritional Information (per serving):
Calories: 192
Fat: 8.8g
Carbohydrates: 29.1g
Fiber: 5.7g
Protein: 2.4g
Sodium: 2mg

Banana Oat Cookies

Servings: *12*

Ingredients:
2 ripe bananas, mashed
1 cup rolled oats
1/4 cup chopped walnuts
1/4 cup raisins
1 tsp vanilla extract

Directions:
1. Preheat oven to 350°F.
2. In a mixing bowl, combine mashed bananas, oats, walnuts, raisins, and vanilla extract.
3. Drop spoonfuls of the mixture onto a baking sheet. Bake for 15-20 minutes or until the edges are golden brown.

Nutritional Information (per serving - 2 cookies):
Calories: 143
Fat: 5.6g
Carbohydrates: 22.5g
Fiber: 3.1g
Protein: 3.5g

Sodium: 2mg

Chocolate Avocado Pudding

Servings: *2*

Ingredients:
1 avocado, pitted and peeled
1/4 cup unsweetened cocoa powder
1/4 cup honey
1 tsp vanilla extract
1/4 cup unsweetened almond milk

Directions:
1. In a food processor, blend avocado until smooth.
2. Add cocoa powder, honey, vanilla extract, and almond milk. Blend until smooth.
3. Transfer the mixture to a bowl and refrigerate for at least 1 hour.

Nutritional Information (per serving):
Calories: 269
Fat: 14.4g
Carbohydrates: 41.7g
Fiber: 9.4g
Protein: 5.1g
Sodium: 57mg

Berry Chia Seed Pudding

Servings: *4*

Ingredients:
1 cup unsweetened almond milk
1 cup mixed berries
1/4 cup chia seeds

1 tbsp honey

Directions:
1. Combine all ingredients in a blender and blend until smooth.
2. Pour the mixture into a jar or container and refrigerate overnight. Serve chilled.

Nutritional Information per serving:
Calories: 160
Fat: 11g
Carbohydrates: 17g
Protein: 3g
Sodium: 10mg

Chocolate Avocado Mousse

Servings: *2*

Ingredients:
1 ripe avocado
1/4 cup unsweetened cocoa powder
1/4 cup maple syrup
1/4 cup unsweetened almond milk

Directions:
1. Scoop the avocado into a blender and add the cocoa powder, maple syrup, and almond milk.
2. Blend until smooth and creamy. Serve chilled.

Nutritional information per serving:
Calories: 175
Protein: 3g
Fat: 14g
Carbohydrates: 15g
Fiber: 6g

Sodium: 9mg
Sugar: 6g

Baked Cinnamon Apple Slices

Servings: *4*

Ingredients:
4 medium apples, cored and sliced
1 tsp ground cinnamon
1 tbsp honey

Directions:
1. Preheat the oven to 375°F.
2. Toss the apple slices with cinnamon and honey in a bowl until evenly coated.
3. Arrange the apple slices in a single layer on a baking sheet lined with parchment paper.
4. Bake for 20-25 minutes or until tender and golden brown. Serve warm or chilled.

Nutritional information per serving:
Calories: 98
Protein: 0g
Fat: 0g
Carbohydrates: 26g
Fiber: 4g
Sodium: 1mg
Sugar: 20g

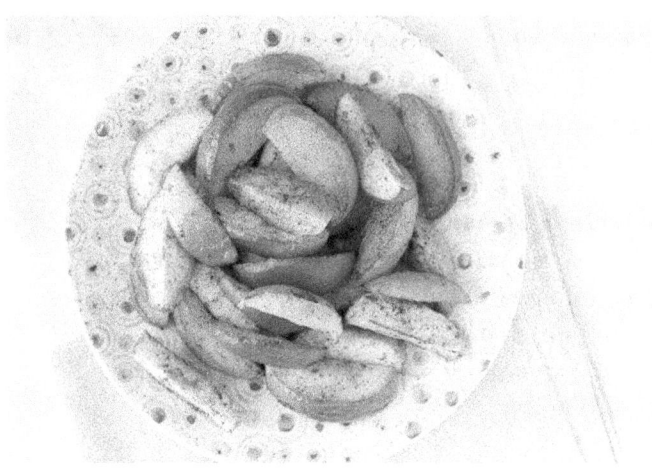

Peanut Butter Banana Ice Cream

Servings: *2*

Ingredients:
2 ripe bananas, sliced and frozen
2 tbsp natural peanut butter
1/4 cup unsweetened almond milk

Directions:
1. Combine the frozen banana slices, peanut butter, and almond milk in a blender.
2. Blend until smooth and creamy.
3. Serve immediately or freeze for later.

Nutritional information per serving:
Calories: 204
Protein: 5g
Fat: 11g
Carbohydrates: 23g
Fiber: 4g
Sodium: 102mg

Sugar: 12g

Carrot Cake Energy Bites

Servings: *12*

Ingredients:
1 cup rolled oats
1/2 cup grated carrots
1/2 cup chopped walnuts
1/4 cup honey
1/4 cup almond butter
1 tsp ground cinnamon
1/4 tsp ground nutmeg

Directions:
1. Combine all ingredients in a mixing bowl and stir until well combined.
2. Roll the mixture into small balls and place on a parchment-lined baking sheet.
3. Refrigerate for 30 minutes or until firm. Serve chilled.

Nutritional information per serving:
Calories: 137
Protein: 3g
Fat: 7g
Carbohydrates: 17g
Fiber: 3g
Sodium: 40mg
Sugar: 10g

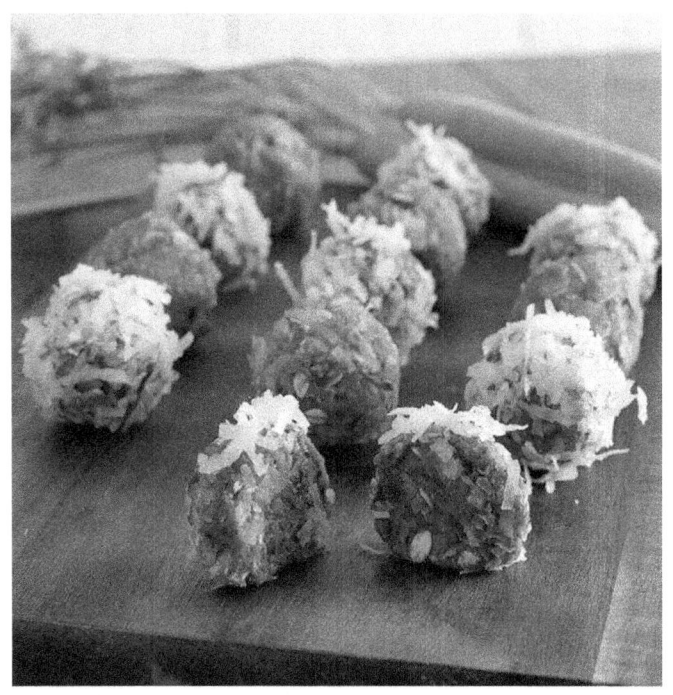

Peach Sorbet:

Servings: *4*

Ingredients:
4 peaches, peeled and diced
1/4 cup honey
1/4 cup water
2 tbsp fresh lemon juice

Directions:
1. Add the diced peaches, honey, water, and lemon juice to a blender and blend until smooth.
2. Pour the mixture into a shallow container and freeze for 4-6 hours, stirring every hour until it reaches a sorbet consistency.
3. Serve and enjoy!

Nutritional Information per serving:
Calories: 108
Fat: 0.5g
Carbohydrates: 28g
Fiber: 2.5g
Protein: 1.5g
Sodium: 0mg

Chocolate Dipped Strawberries:

Servings: *4*

Ingredients:
8-10 large strawberries
1/4 cup dark chocolate chips
1 tsp coconut oil

Directions:
1. Rinse the strawberries and pat dry.
2. In a small bowl, melt the dark chocolate chips and coconut oil in the microwave or on a double boiler.
3. Dip the strawberries in the melted chocolate and place them on a parchment-lined baking sheet.
4. Chill in the refrigerator for 10-15 minutes until the chocolate is set. Serve and enjoy!

Nutritional Information per serving:
Calories: 60
Fat: 3.5g
Carbohydrates: 9g
Fiber: 1.5g
Protein: 1g
Sodium: 1mg

Greek Yogurt and Berry Parfait:

Servings: *2*

Ingredients:
1 cup non-fat Greek yogurt
1/2 cup fresh mixed berries (such as strawberries, blueberries, and raspberries)
2 tbsp honey
1/4 cup granola

Directions:
1. In two small jars or glasses, layer the Greek yogurt, mixed berries, honey, and granola.
2. Repeat the layers until the jars or glasses are full. Serve and enjoy!

Nutritional Information per serving:
Calories: 205
Fat: 3g
Carbohydrates: 38g
Fiber: 3.5g
Protein: 12g
Sodium: 63mg

Tips for satisfying your sweet tooth without excess sugar

Satisfying your sweet tooth can be a challenge when trying to maintain a healthy diet, especially if you're trying to limit your sugar intake. However, there are plenty of ways to enjoy sweet treats without overloading on sugar. By making a few simple swaps and adjustments, you can still indulge in your favorite sweets while staying on track with your health goals. In this section, we'll explore some tips and tricks for satisfying your sweet tooth without excess sugar, so you can enjoy your favorite desserts in moderation

Choose naturally sweet foods: Instead of reaching for a candy bar, try satisfying your sweet cravings with naturally sweet foods such as fruits, dried fruits, or sweet vegetables like carrots.

Use spices: Adding spices such as cinnamon, nutmeg, or ginger to your food can help satisfy your sweet tooth without adding any sugar.

Opt for dark chocolate: Dark chocolate contains less sugar than milk chocolate and has more antioxidants, which can be beneficial for your health. Just make sure to choose a variety with a high percentage of cocoa.

Try natural sweeteners: Natural sweeteners such as honey, maple syrup, or stevia can be used in moderation to sweeten foods and drinks without adding refined sugar.

Make your own desserts: By making your own desserts, you can control the amount of sugar you add and opt for healthier ingredients like whole grains, fruits, and nuts.

Be mindful of portion sizes: Even healthier sweet treats should be consumed in moderation. Pay attention to portion sizes to avoid overindulging in sugar.

Chapter 7

Eating Out on the DASH Diet

Eating out can be a challenge when you're trying to follow a specific diet like the DASH diet, which focuses on whole, unprocessed foods and limits sodium and added sugars. But with a little planning and strategy, it's possible to enjoy a meal out while sticking to your dietary goals. In this chapter, we discuss ideas for navigating menus and making healthy choices when eating out on the DASH diet.

Strategies for sticking to the DASH Diet while eating out

Plan ahead: Before going out to eat, research the restaurant and look at the menu online. Choose a restaurant that offers healthy options and avoid those that are known for high-calorie or high-fat dishes.

Make special requests: Don't be afraid to ask for substitutions or special requests to make your meal healthier. For example, ask for dressings and sauces on the side, or substitute fries for a side salad.

Watch your portions: Many restaurants serve portions that are much larger than necessary. Consider splitting an entrée with a friend, or ask for a to-go box and take half of your meal home.

Stick to the basics: Choose simple dishes that are grilled, baked, or steamed instead of fried or sautéed. Opt for lean protein sources like fish or chicken, and load up on vegetables.

Be mindful of drinks: Sugary drinks like soda and fruit juice can add a significant amount of calories and sugar to your meal. Stick to water, unsweetened tea, or other low-calorie drinks.

By following these strategies, you can still enjoy eating out while staying on track with the DASH Diet.

Healthy options to look for on restaurant menus

When trying to stick to the DASH diet while eating out, it can be a challenge to find healthy options on restaurant menus. However, with a bit of planning and knowledge, it's possible to make healthy choices when dining out
.

One of the first things to consider is the type of restaurant you are going to. If possible, look for restaurants that offer fresh, whole foods and avoid fast food and chain restaurants that tend to serve highly processed and high sodium meals.

When looking at the menu, start by focusing on dishes that are centered around vegetables, fruits, and lean proteins such as grilled fish or chicken. Look for menu items that are steamed, roasted, grilled, or baked rather than fried or sautéed.

Don't be afraid to ask questions or make special requests to accommodate your dietary needs. Many restaurants are willing to accommodate special requests such as substituting vegetables for fries or leaving off sauces and dressings.

It's also important to pay attention to portion sizes. Many restaurants serve portions that are much larger than what is recommended for a healthy diet. Consider sharing an entrée with a friend or taking home half of your meal for later.

Lastly, be mindful of drinks and desserts. Many beverages and desserts are high in sugar and calories. Opt for water, unsweetened tea, or sparkling water instead of sugary drinks, and consider splitting a dessert with a friend or skipping it altogether.

By following these strategies, you can enjoy eating out while still maintaining your DASH diet goals.

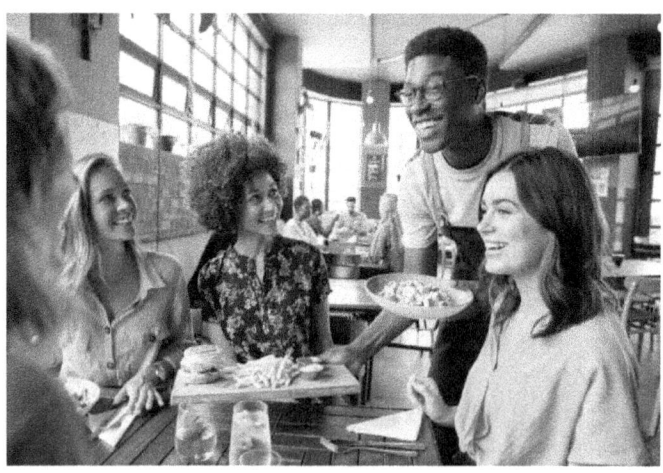

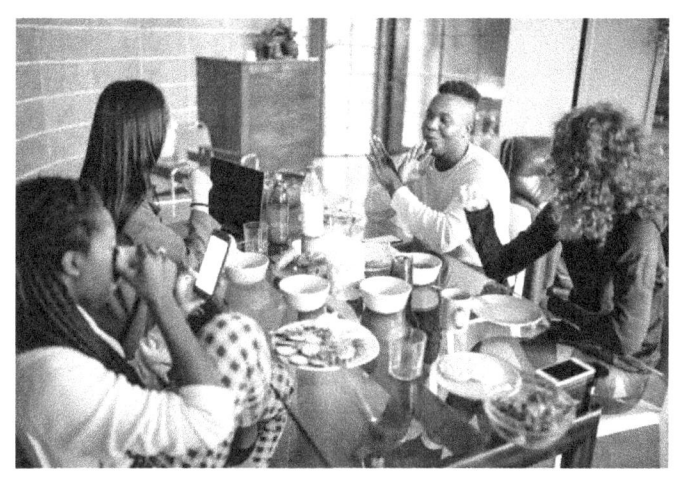

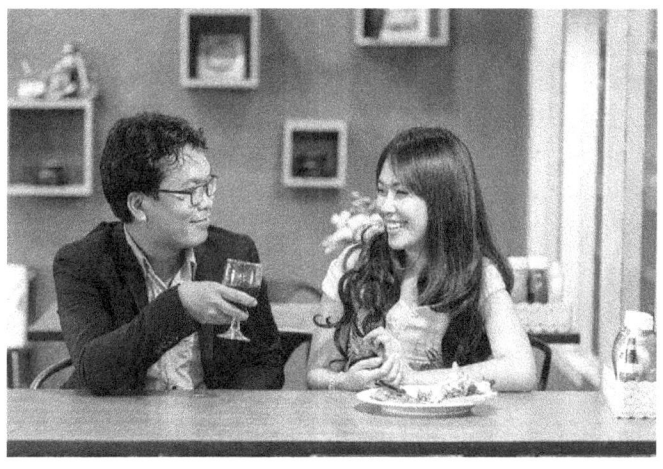

Chapter 8

Exercise and Lifestyle Tips for Lowering Blood Pressure

High blood pressure, also known as hypertension, is a common health concern affecting millions of people worldwide. It can increase the risk of heart disease, stroke, and other health complications if left uncontrolled. While medication is often recommended to control high blood pressure, making lifestyle changes can also be beneficial in reducing blood pressure levels. Regular exercise, healthy eating habits, and stress management techniques are just a few examples of lifestyle changes that can help lower blood pressure. In this section, we will discuss some exercise and lifestyle tips that can aid in the management of high blood pressure

Incorporating physical activity into a busy schedule

Incorporating physical activity into a busy schedule can be challenging, but it's essential for lowering blood pressure and improving overall health. Here are some tips to help you get moving:

Schedule it in: Treat exercise like any other appointment and add it to your calendar. Plan your week ahead of time and make sure to include time for physical activity.

Get creative: Exercise doesn't have to mean hitting the gym or going for a run. Find fun and creative ways to get moving, like dancing, hiking, or playing a sport.

Multitask: Incorporate exercise into your daily routine by walking or biking to work, taking the stairs instead of the elevator, or doing squats while brushing your teeth.

Find a workout buddy: Enlist a friend or family member to join you for workouts. This can help keep you motivated and make exercise more enjoyable.

Start small: Don't feel like you have to jump into a rigorous exercise routine right away. Start small by incorporating short walks or light stretching into your day, and gradually work your way up to more intense workouts.

Remember, any physical activity is better than none. Even small changes can make a big difference in lowering your blood pressure and improving your overall health.

Managing stress and getting enough sleep for optimal health

Stress and sleep are essential factors in maintaining overall health and well-being, and they can significantly impact blood pressure. Stress triggers the body's "fight or flight" response, which can cause blood pressure to increase temporarily.

However, chronic stress can lead to sustained high blood pressure, which can increase the risk of heart disease, stroke, and other health problems. Adequate sleep, on the other hand, can help regulate blood pressure and promote overall health.

There are several strategies for managing stress and getting enough sleep, including engaging in relaxation techniques such as meditation, deep breathing, and yoga. Regular physical activity can also help reduce stress and improve sleep quality. Additionally, establishing a consistent sleep schedule, avoiding caffeine and alcohol before bedtime, and creating a relaxing sleep environment can all contribute to better sleep habits.

It's important to prioritize stress management and sleep in your overall health routine. By making small, sustainable changes in your lifestyle, you can help reduce your risk of high blood pressure and other health problems. Consult with your healthcare provider for personalized recommendations and guidance.

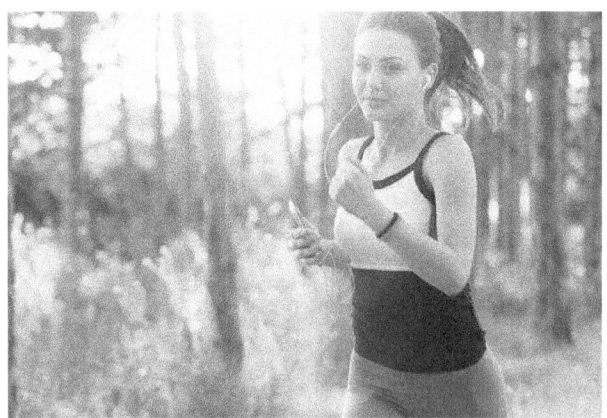

Conclusion

In conclusion, the DASH diet is a well-researched and effective way to lower blood pressure and improve overall health. By focusing on whole foods, limiting processed foods, and reducing sodium intake, individuals can see significant improvements in their blood pressure and overall well-being. In addition to following the DASH diet, incorporating regular physical activity, managing stress, and getting enough sleep are also important components of a healthy lifestyle. With these tips and strategies, individuals can make sustainable changes to their diet and lifestyle to achieve their health goals and improve their quality of life.

Chapter 9

Recap of the benefits of the DASH Diet for busy professionals

As a recap, the DASH Diet is a flexible and healthy eating plan that emphasizes whole, nutrient-dense foods while limiting processed and high-sugar foods. Busy professionals can benefit from the DASH Diet by increasing their intake of fruits, vegetables, lean proteins, and whole grains, which can help improve heart health, lower blood pressure, and reduce the risk of chronic diseases.

In addition, meal planning and prepping can help busy professionals stay on track with the DASH Diet, and incorporating physical activity and stress-management techniques can enhance the overall benefits of this healthy lifestyle approach. By making small changes to their diet and lifestyle, busy professionals can prioritize their health and well-being, leading to improved energy levels, productivity, and overall quality of life.

Tips for staying motivated and on track with your diet and lifestyle changes.

Staying motivated and on track with diet and lifestyle changes can be challenging, especially for busy professionals. However, it is essential to maintain motivation to achieve long-term health and wellness goals. Here are some tips to help you stay motivated and on track:

Set specific, achievable goals: Setting specific goals can help you stay focused and motivated. Make sure your goals are achievable and realistic.

Celebrate your successes: Celebrate your successes, no matter how small they may seem. Recognizing your progress can help you stay motivated and positive.

Find a support system: Having a support system can help keep you accountable and motivated. Joining a support group or working with a dietitian or personal trainer can be beneficial.

Keep a food and exercise journal: Keeping track of what you eat and your physical activity can help you stay on track and identify areas where you may need to make changes.

Make it fun: Find ways to make healthy eating and exercise fun. Try new healthy recipes or incorporate activities you enjoy into your workout routine.

Stay positive: Stay positive and don't beat yourself up if you slip up. Remember, each day is a new day, and every small step counts towards reaching your goals.

By incorporating these tips into your daily routine, you can stay motivated and on track with your diet and lifestyle changes, ultimately achieving better health and wellness.

CHECK OUT MY OTHER BOOKS

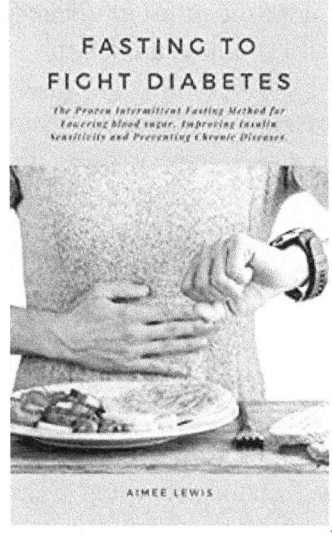
Fighting to Fight Diabetes

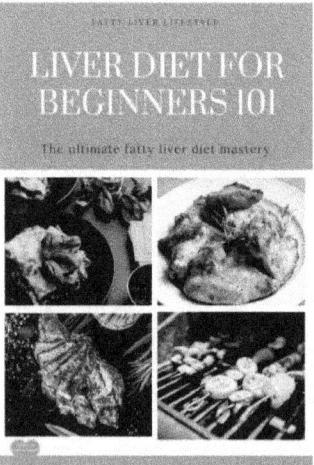
Liver Diet for Beginners 101

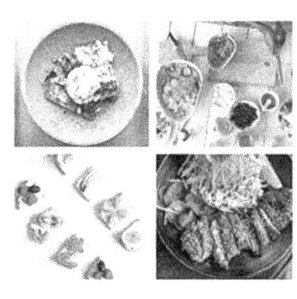

HEART FRIENDLY
RECIPES MASTERY

*Easy-to-prepare, heart-friendly recipes for
the busy 9-5 worker*

BY CHEF TIMET LEWIS

Heart Friendly Recipes Mastery

Request for Review

If you found this book beneficial, I would appreciate it if you could provide an honest review on the Amazon website. Your help is greatly appreciated and makes a significant difference.

I personally read all of the reviews in order to gainrealistic feedback on how I can make adjustments and modifications that will help future readers. It's really simple to leave a review if you feel so inclined. All you have to do is go to the Amazon page for this book and click on the "leave a customer review" button - this will take you directly to the review section.

I am grateful for your assistance.

Sincere Regards

Aimee

THE END